Study Guide for

RADIOLOGY for the
Dental Professional

Study Guide for

RADIOLOGY for the
Dental Professional

HERBERT H. FROMMER, BA, DDS, FACD

Diplomat of the American Board of Oral and Maxillofacial Radiology
Professor Emeritus of Radiology
New York University
College of Dentistry
New York, New York

JEANINE J. STABULAS-SAVAGE, RDH, BS, MPH

Assistant Clinical Professor of Radiology
New York University
College of Dentistry
New York, New York

MOSBY
ELSEVIER

3251 Riverport Lane
St. Louis, Missouri 63043

STUDY GUIDE FOR RADIOLOGY FOR THE DENTAL
PROFESSIONAL, NINTH EDITION

ISBN: 978-0-323-06399-9

ISBN: 978-0-323-06399-9

Vice President and Publisher: Linda Duncan
Executive Editor: John Dolan
Developmental Editor: Joslyn Dumas
Publishing Services Manager: Julie Eddy
Project Manager: Marquita Parker
Designer: Paula Catalano

Printed in United States

Last digit is the print number: 9 8 7 6 5 4 3 2 1

Preface

This study guide is intended to accompany the ninth edition of the textbook *Radiology for the Dental Professional*. The ninth edition of this study guide includes additional questions not included in the previous editions.

Each chapter in the study guide relates to a corresponding chapter in the textbook and stresses the essential information of the chapter through the use of definitions, short essays (comprehension), matching questions, illustrations, completion, and multiple choice questions. The answers for the matching, illustrations, completion, and multiple choice questions are available in the instructor's section of the Evolve resource site.

Educational objectives are included at the beginning of each chapter to help the students focus on the material and concepts they are expected to learn and how this information is to be applied in the dental clinical setting.

The following suggestions will help students use this study guide to identify strengths and weaknesses.

1. Review the contents of each chapter before you attempt to do the exercise. Do not treat the questions individually and then refer to the text for the correct answer. Deal with the chapter's subject matter as a whole, since many of the questions are interrelated. This is a learning exercise meant to help you learn the material presented in the textbook, not an examination for grades.
2. Remember that the same subject matter may be repeated in different question forms in each chapter or other chapters, since the material overlaps. The subjects of the questions are not in the same order as they appear in the textbook, so don't expect to find a question in order for every page.
3. Read each question and study each illustration carefully before answering. You may know the answer or you may arrive at the correct answer by knowing which answers are incorrect.

This study guide is designed so that the pages can be easily removed, submitted if required, and placed in the student's notebook with the corresponding lecture notes.

Herbert H. Frommer
Jeanine J. Stabulas-Savage

Contents

Ionizing Radiation and Basic Principles of X-Ray Generation

Educational Objectives

After reading Chapter 1 of the textbook and completing this exercise, the student will

1. Understand the nature and production of ionizing radiation and the history of x-rays.
2. Understand the generation of x-rays in the dental x-ray tube.
3. Be able to apply these concepts and principles to clinical radiography.

I. Definitions

Define/explain the following terms.

1. Atom _____

_____

2. Binding energy _____

_____

3. Bremsstrahlung _____

_____

4. Electromagnetic spectrum _____

_____

5. Energy wave _____

_____

6. Frequency _____

_____

7. Hittoft-Crookes tube _____

_____

8. Ionization _____

_____

9. Isotope _____

_____

10. Photon energy _____

_____

11. Radiation _____

_____

12. Radioactive _____

_____

13. Thermionic emission effect _____

_____

14. Wavelength _____

_____

15. X-rays _____

_____

II. Comprehension Exercise

1. Explain the differences and similarities between radio waves and x-rays and their significance in dental radiology.

2. Explain why the dental x-ray machine is said to be "inefficient" in the production of x-radiation.

3. What is the source of the heat produced in the dental x-ray tube?

4. Explain the difference between duty rating and duty cycle.

5. Compare the binding energy of the various shells of an atom.

6. Clarify the difference between characteristic x-rays and Bremsstrahlung x-rays.

7. Explain the function of the molybdenum focusing cup.

8. What accounts for ionizing radiation's potential to cause harmful biologic effects? Explain.

9. Cite the reasons for using tungsten as the material for the target in the dental x-ray tube.

10. Explain the difference between the filament and the high-tension circuit in the dental x-ray tube.

11. Describe the difference between the on/off switch and the exposure switch.

12. Compare the source of electrons in the original x-ray tubes with today's tubes.

13. List at least five properties of x-radiation as evidenced in dental radiographic procedures.

14. State the significance of the high-tension circuit in the production of x-rays in dentistry.

15. What is the relationship between the "wavelength" of a specific radiation and its ability to penetrate opaque structures?

III. Matching

Match the items in *Column A* with the appropriate items in *Column B*.

Column A

_____ 1. electrons
_____ 2. binding energy
_____ 3. focal spot
_____ 4. particulate radiation
_____ 5. Crookes tube
_____ 6. unit of x-ray exposure
_____ 7. 70 kVp or above
_____ 8. protons
_____ 9. short wavelengths
_____ 10. ionization
_____ 11. focusing cup
_____ 12. unstable isotopes
_____ 13. thermionic emission effect
_____ 14. shells
_____ 15. atomic mass

Column B

a. fixed orbits
b. cathode
c. gamma rays
d. number of protons
e. electron cloud
f. anode
g. tungsten filament
h. negative charge
i. number of neutrons
j. beta particles
k. characteristic x-rays
l. positive charge
m. x-rays
n. K shell
o. Roentgen
p. roentgen
q. loss of an electron

IV. Illustrations

1. (Figure 1-1) Label the components in this diagram of an atom.

a.

b.

c.

d.

e.

f.

2. (Figure 1-2) Identify the lettered components in this diagram of the dental x-ray tube and list the function of each.

Component	Function
a.	
b.	
c.	
d.	
e.	
f.	
g.	
h.	
i.	
j.	
k.	

3. Provide a schematic drawing of the composition of matter.

4. (Figure 1-3) In this schematic drawing of dental x-rays, which x-ray, A or B:

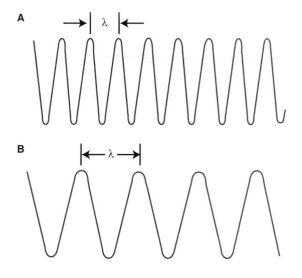

a. has the longest wavelength? _____
b. has the most energy? _____
c. has the higher frequency? _____
d. would be more penetrating? _____

5. Draw a diagram of the Bremsstrahlung reaction at the tungsten target.

V. Complete These Statements

1. An example of particulate radiation is
   _____,
   _____,
   _____,
   _____, or
   _____.

2. The effect of electromagnetic radiation on living organisms varies depending on the
   _____.

3. The amount of energy contained in electromagnetic radiation is determined by their _____ and
   _____.

4. Electric current within the dental x-ray tube flows from a
   _____ pole to a
   _____ pole.

5. Patients undergoing cancer therapy may receive radiation treatment from
   _____.

6. When atoms have the same atomic number but different atomic mass numbers, they are called
   _____.

7. A _____ is the smallest particle of a substance that retains the properties of the substance.

8. Individual units of radiation energy are referred to as _____.

9. In the dental x-ray machine the amount of energy produced at the anode as heat is
   _____%.

10. X-rays can affect a photographic emulsion that, when processed, produces
    _____.

11. The _____ refers to the number of consecutive seconds a machine can be operated before overheating.

12. Particulate radiations most commonly are emitted from radioactive substances called
    _____.

13. Two examples of electromagnetic radiation are _____ and _____.

14. The three basic elements of an x-ray tube needed to produce x-rays are:
    (1) _____,
    (2) _____, and
    (3) _____.

15. The milliamperage dial controls the _____ of electrons that "boil off" the tungsten filament.

VI. Multiple Choice

Select the best answer.

1. Which of the following occurs at 70 kVp or higher and accounts for a very small part of the x-rays produced in the dental x-ray machine?
   a. Bremsstrahlung radiation
   b. Compton scatter
   c. characteristic radiation
   d. coherent scatter
   e. photoelectron interaction

2. Which of the following delineates where the thermionic emission effect takes place?
   a. tungsten target
   b. focal area
   c. tungsten filament of the anode
   d. tungsten filament at the cathode
   e. step-down transformer

3. The person accredited with the initial discovery of x-rays is
   a. Dr. Otto Walkhoff
   b. William D. Coolidge
   c. Wilhelm Conrad Roentgen
   d. Thomas Alva Edison
   e. Dr. C. Edmond Kells

4. You turn on the dental x-ray machine in the morning for your first patient. In doing so, you
   a. activate the high-tension circuit
   b. heat the anode
   c. activate the filament circuit
   d. turn on the step-up transformer
   e. produce x-rays

5. Which of the following electrons has the greatest binding energy?
   a. N shell electrons
   b. M shell electrons
   c. L shell electrons
   d. K shell electrons
   e. None of the above

6. X-rays are generated when a stream of electrons traveling from one side of a vacuum tube is stopped suddenly by its impact on the
   a. filament cup
   b. tungsten target of the anode
   c. tungsten target of the cathode
   d. focusing cup
   e. copper stem

7. Which of the following does not occur when the high voltage circuit is activated?
   a. The x-ray machine produces an audible and visible signal.
   b. Electrons travel from the filament to the target.
   c. Heat is produced.
   d. Electrons produced at the cathode fire across the tube and hit the target.
   e. X-rays are produced at the filament.

8. All of the following are examples of electromagnetic radiation *except*
   a. x-rays
   b. beta rays
   c. gamma rays
   d. microwaves
   e. light waves

9. Which of the following statements are *not* true concerning radioactive substances?
   a. They are utilized in cancer therapy.
   b. They are unstable elements.
   c. They produce high-energy waves.
   d. They are utilized to produce an image in dental radiography.
   e. All of the above are true.

10. Which of the following is incorrect?
    a. X-rays have no charge.
    b. X-rays have no weight.
    c. X-rays travel at the speed of sound.
    d. X-rays have short wavelengths.
    e. X-rays cause ionization in tissues.

11. The dental x-ray tube is said to be "inefficient" because
    a. energy flows from the negative to the positive pole
    b. 1% of the energy produced is x-radiation
    c. the radiation produced is x-radiation
    d. it has a duty rating and a duty cycle
    e. it can overheat if used too frequently

12. As a result of the multiple Bremsstrahlung reactions,
    a. a heterogeneous x-ray spectrum is produced
    b. the succeeding x-rays produced will have less energy
    c. the later x-rays produced have less penetrating ability
    d. the wavelengths are different
    e. All of the above are valid statements.

13. Which of the following has the ability to affect living organisms?
    a. supervoltage x-rays
    b. microwaves
    c. magnetic resonance imaging
    d. electric waves
    e. ultrasonic waves

14. To prevent the x-ray tube and its components from overheating,
    a. each machine has a duty cycle and a duty rating
    b. the milliamperage setting should not exceed 15
    c. rotating anodes are utilized in extraoral radiography
    d. the copper sleeve surrounds the target
    e. All of the above are true.

15. The radiation produced at the atomic level in dental radiography is predominantly as a result of
    a. characteristic radiation
    b. radioactivity
    c. gamma rays
    d. Bremsstrahlung
    e. total energy loss

VII. True/False

Select whether each statement is true (**T**) or false (**F**). Circle the correct answer.

1. The focusing cup is found at the cathode. **T/F**
2. Bremsstrahlung radiation is the main source of radiation in the dental tube. **T/F**
3. X-rays are weightless. **T/F**
4. Ten percent of all reactions in the tube produce heat. **T/F**
5. X-rays are a type of ionizing radiation. **T/F**

Chapter

2

The Dental X-Ray Machine

Educational Objectives

After reading Chapter 2 of the textbook and completing this exercise, the student will
1. Understand the function of the dental x-ray machine.
2. Understand the function of the settings in the dental x-ray unit, the variables of the control panel, and the properties of the x-ray beam.
3. Be able to apply these concepts and principles to clinical radiography.

I. Definitions

Define/explain the following terms.

1. Alternating current _____

    _____

2. Central ray _____

    _____

3. Collimation _____

    _____

4. Direct current _____

    _____

5. Electric current _____

    _____

6. Filtration _____

    _____

7. Half-value layer (HVL) _____

    _____

8. Inherent filtration _____

    _____

9. Rectangular collimation _____

    _____

10. Rectification _____

_____

11. Scatter radiation _____

_____

12. Transformer _____

_____

13. Total filtration _____

_____

14. Useful beam _____

_____

15. Voltage _____

_____

II. Comprehension Exercise

1. Explain the difference between filtration and collimation of the x-ray beam. What are the clinical consequences of each?

2. Explain the difference between milliamperage and kilovoltage in the dental x-ray machine. What is the clinical significance of each?

3. Explain the concept of milliampere seconds (mAs).

4. Explain why exposure times are best expressed in impulses rather than in fractions of seconds.

5. What is rectangular collimation? Why is it important?

6. Do all x-ray photons at the anode of the x-ray tube have the same energy? Why? If not, what is done to correct this situation?

7. Explain why the use of an alternating current produces a heterogeneous x-ray beam.

8. What is the ideal size and shape of an intraoral x-ray beam?

9. What are the types of transformers used in the dental x-ray machine, and what is their function?

10. Why are electronic timers recommended for contemporary use as opposed to the utilization of the old mechanical timers?

11. What factors determine the intensity of the x-ray beam? Explain your answer.

12. Why is the half-value layer a more appropriate means of describing beam quality and penetration than kilovoltage?

13. What factors are used to determine the milliampere seconds required at a given kilovoltage? What is the clinical significance of using a higher milliamperage and a shorter exposure time?

14. What are the federal regulation specifications regarding total filtration of the x-ray beam at various kilovoltage settings?

15. Why would a change to rectangular collimation increase the incidence of collimator cutoff? How could this change be achieved without evidence of an increase in this exposure error?

III. Matching

Match the items in *Column A* with the appropriate items in *Column B*.

Column A

_____ 1. lead diaphragm
_____ 2. impulse
_____ 3. filtration
_____ 4. ampere
_____ 5. useful beam
_____ 6. rectangular collimation
_____ 7. electricity
_____ 8. quantity of x-rays
_____ 9. cycle
_____ 10. pointed cone
_____ 11. position-indicating device (PID)
_____ 12. rectification
_____ 13. half-value layer (HVL)
_____ 14. mechanical timers
_____ 15. quality of x-rays

Column B

a. removes long wavelengths
b. collimating device
c. x-ray beam after filtration and collimation
d. kilovoltage control
e. open-ended cylinder/rectangle
f. scatter radiation
g. x-ray beam penetration
h. energy source for radiation production
i. ⅙₀ second margin of error
j. comparable to #2 size film packet
k. milliamperage control
l. lead
m. ⅙₀ of a second
n. electrical current reversal blocking
o. x-rays
p. measures electrical current flow
q. flow and reversal of electrical current

IV. Illustrations

1. (Figure 2-1) Identify the lettered components in this diagram of the tube head of a dental x-ray machine.

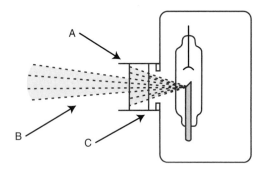

a.

b.

c.

2. (Figure 2-2) Outline in red the areas that would be exposed by the x-ray beam that do not contribute to the image when using circular collimation. Do the same in blue for rectangular collimation.

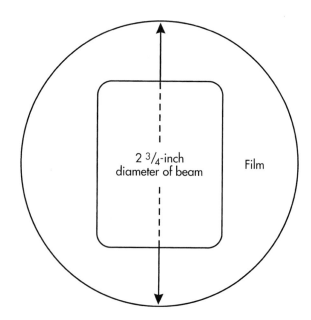

2 ¾-inch diameter of beam

Film

3. (Figure 2-3) Explain how this diagram of alternating current shows the effect of dental x-rays.

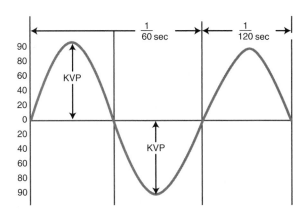

_____

_____

_____

4. (Figure 2-4) Indicate where characteristic x-rays are shown on this diagram.

5. (Figure 2-5) What is the remedy for the condition illustrated on this diagram?

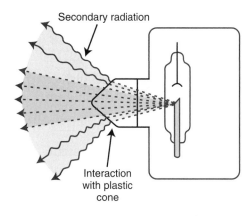

_____

_____

_____

V. Complete These Statements

1. The closed-end pointed cone should not be used as a PID because it creates

   _____.

2. The diameter of the x-ray beam for intraoral radiographs, measured at the face, should be no larger than

   _____.

3. Filtration of the dental x-ray beam is necessary because the beam contains

   _____,

   _____ x-rays.

4. In a dental x-ray machine operating at 75 kVp, the required total filtration would be _____.

5. If the kilovoltage is increased with no other change in exposure factors, the resultant film will appear

   _____ and

   _____.

6. Limiting the size of the x-ray beam is called _____.

7. On the control panel of the x-ray machine the penetrating power of the x-ray beam is controlled by the _____ dial and the number of x-rays produced is controlled by the _____ dial.

8. In real time, 20 impulses represent _____ second.

9. Limiting the size of the x-ray beam to just slightly larger than the actual size of the film packet is done by using _____.

10. Various new dental x-ray machine models are designed to supply _____ rectification in which the portion of the alternating cycle is reversed.

11. The term _____ is used to denote the maximum voltage that is described by the sine wave that plots the alternation of the current.

12. Some dental x-ray machines have preset fixed milliamperage choices, usually at _____, _____, or _____ mA.

13. The x-ray at the midpoint of the beam is known as the _____ ray.

14. Radiation protection codes in many states require the use of lead-lined, _____ PIDs.

15. The three parameters of the dental x-ray beam that are adjusted from the control panel are (1) _____, (2) _____, and (3) _____.

VI. Multiple Choice

Select the best answer.

1. Filters are used in the x-ray beam to
   a. increase density
   b. reduce density
   c. reduce exposure time
   d. correct the size of the beam
   e. reduce patient radiation dose

2. Proper collimation of the x-ray beam for film size and focal-film distance will
   a. improve image definition
   b. increase radiographic contrast
   c. increase the intensity of the central beam
   d. increase secondary radiation
   e. reduce primary radiation

3. The best way to describe the penetration of an x-ray beam is by its
   a. half-value layer
   b. kilovoltage
   c. milliamperage
   d. rad output
   e. roentgen output

4. The milliampere control dial on the dental x-ray machine
   a. regulates the step-up transformer
   b. determines the penetration of the x-ray
   c. regulates the quality of the radiation
   d. regulates the quantity of the radiation
   e. regulates scatter radiation

5. You have taken a radiograph of a patient with a large skeletal build. The resulting image does not show the bone trabeculation well and appears to be underpenetrated. The adjustment that should be made for the retake is
   a. reduce the mA
   b. reduce the exposure time
   c. increase the kVp
   d. reduce the kVp
   e. check the processing solution temperature

6. In taking the radiograph, you did not center the beam on the film in the patient's mouth. The resulting film will show
   a. fogging
   b. overlapping
   c. elongation
   d. collimator cutoff (cone cutting)
   e. foreshortening

7. The dental x-ray machine in your office operates at 90 kVp and thus is required to have a total filtration of
   a. 2.75 inches of aluminum
   b. 2.5 inches of aluminum
   c. 2.0 mm of aluminum
   d. 2.5 mm of aluminum
   e. 1.5 mm of aluminum

8. The radiation inspector comes to your office and tells you that your x-ray beam has an HVL of 1.00 mm of aluminum. You should
   a. feel assured that the beam meets the recommended standards
   b. be concerned because of the unnecessary secondary radiation to your patients
   c. be concerned because the beam is too penetrating
   d. add more filtration
   e. use a different PID

9. The x-ray beam from a conventional dental machine is
   a. a continuous beam
   b. a convergent beam
   c. a continuous divergent beam
   d. a pulsating divergent beam
   e. none of the above

10. Using a 16-inch focal-film distance, the diameter of the beam measured at the patient's face should be no larger than
    a. 1 inch
    b. 3 inches
    c. 2.75 cm
    d. 1.5 cm
    e. 2.75 inches

11. For x-ray timers calibrated in impulses, how many impulses are there in a second?
    a. 10
    b. 30
    c. 60
    d. 120
    e. 15

12. The intensity of the beam is affected by the
    a. kilovolt peak
    b. milliamperage
    c. exposure time
    d. focal-film distance
    e. all of the above

13. How many times per second is the polarity reversed in a dental x-ray machine operating on an alternating current?
    a. 30
    b. 15
    c. 60
    d. 45
    e. none of the above

14. The high-voltage circuit in the dental x-ray machine requires voltage in the range of 65,000 to 100,000, which is achieved by the use of the
    a. step-up transformer
    b. high-tension circuit
    c. autotransformer
    d. low-tension circuit
    e. step-down transformer

15. Which of the following materials is most resistant to x-radiation?
    a. copper
    b. molybdenum
    c. tungsten
    d. lead
    e. aluminum

VII. True/False

Select whether each statement is true (**T**) or false (**F**). Circle the correct answer.

1. Milliamperage determines the speed of the electrons. **T/F**
2. The dental x-ray tube is self-rectified. **T/F**
3. The dental x-ray beam is homogeneous. **T/F**
4. Kilovoltage determines the penetration of the beam. **T/F**
5. In 60-cycle alternating current, there are 30 pulses of x-ray per second. **T/F**

Image Formation

Educational Objectives

After reading Chapter 3 of the textbook and completing this exercise, the student will
1. Understand the principles of image formation and the factors that influence the image in dental radiography.
2. Be able to apply these principles to the clinical situation in taking proper radiographs with the least amount of radiation exposure to the patient.

I. Definitions

Define/explain the following terms.

1. Actual focal area _____

   _____

2. Bisecting-angle technique _____

   _____

3. Blurred image _____

   _____

4. Contrast _____

   _____

5. Detail _____

   _____

6. Effective focal area _____

   _____

7. Film density _____

   _____

8. Film fog _____

   _____

9. Focal-film distance (FFD) _____

   _____

10. Illuminator _____

_____

11. Image magnification _____

_____

12. Inverse square law _____

_____

13. Long-scale contrast _____

_____

14. Object density _____

_____

15. Object-film distance (OFD) _____

_____

16. Paralleling technique _____

_____

17. Penumbra _____

_____

18. Recessed tube (recessed target) _____

_____

19. Short-scale contrast _____

_____

20. Umbra _____

_____

II. Comprehension Exercise

1. What factors determine film contrast?

2. What is the ideal technique and setting for viewing radiographs?

3. What is the importance of the target area size?

4. What are the factors that influence image detail?

5. What is the ideal relationship in intraoral radiography of the central ray, tooth, and film? Can this be achieved?

6. Does the patient receive a larger radiation dose with the longer exposures in the 16-inch FFD technique than with a comparable radiograph using the 8-inch FFD technique?

7. Explain how an increased FFD compensates for an increased OFD while using the paralleling radiographic exposure technique?

8. Why is there less image magnification with a 12-inch FFD than with an 8-inch FFD?

9. Name the possible types of movement that could occur in dental radiography and their respective consequences.

10. What are the advantages of using a 90-kVp setting rather than a 65-kVp setting?

11. Why is an FFD of greater than 16 inches not recommended?

12. What criteria must be met in terms of definition, image enlargement, and distortion to produce the "ideal radiograph" of a tooth or other structure?

13. What factors determine object contrast?

14. What would the result be of using an FFD of less than 8 inches?

15. What is meant by the concept of a recessed tube (recessed target)? What is its purpose?

16. Explain the difference between long-scale and short-scale film contrast. How are they determined?

17. When changing from an 8-inch FFD to a 16-inch FFD, what changes, if any, must be made to the collimator?

18. Explain the inverse square law. Give two clinical applications of its use.

19. What are the advantages of the 16-inch FFD technique over the 8-inch technique?

20. What is the ultimate goal of dental radiography regardless of the type of imaging system used?

III. Matching

Match the items in *Column A* with the appropriate items in *Column B*.

Column A

_____ 1. blurred image
_____ 2. tooth-film position
_____ 3. right-angle technique
_____ 4. long-scale contrast
_____ 5. inverse square law
_____ 6. penumbra
_____ 7. radiolucent
_____ 8. illuminator
_____ 9. focal area size
_____ 10. short-scale contrast
_____ 11. radiopaque
_____ 12. thin film
_____ 13. umbra
_____ 14. dense film
_____ 15. density

Column B

a. unsharpness
b. degree of blackness
c. high contrast
d. paralleling technique
e. x-ray intensity
f. viewbox
g. overexposed
h. white (LIGHT) areas
i. sharpness
j. object-film distance
k. patient movement
l. secondary radiation
m. underexposure
n. bisecting method
o. low contrast
p. black (DARK) areas
q. detail

IV. Illustrations

1. (Figure 3-1) Which tube head (used to produce the same film) will result in greater radiation exposure to the patient: A or B? Or would the patient receive the same amount of radiation exposure?

_____

_____

_____

A

B

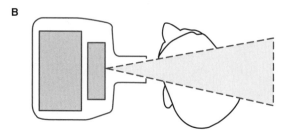

2. (Figure 3-2) If the exposure time for position A of the focal area is 20 impulses at 65 kVp and 10 mA, what would the exposure time be at position B, with the same kVp and mA, to produce the same radiograph?

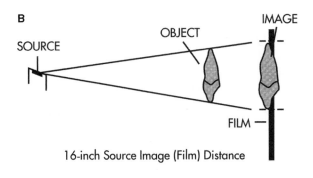

A

SOURCE

OBJECT ─┤ IMAGE
└ FILM

8-inch Source Image (Film) Distance

B

SOURCE

IMAGE

OBJECT

FILM ─

16-inch Source Image (Film) Distance

_____

_____

_____

3. (Figure 3-3) In this diagram of the bisecting technique how would you describe the image that is produced?

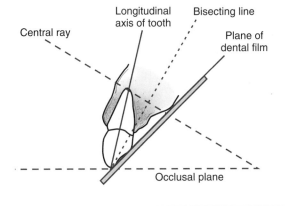

Central ray

Longitudinal axis of tooth   Bisecting line

Plane of dental film

Occlusal plane

_____

_____

_____

4. (Figure 3-4) Label the focal-film, object-film, and focal-object distances.

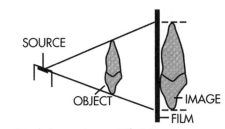

Object

Focal point

Film

A
B
C

a.

b.

c.

5. (Figure 3-5) In this five-step density scale, between which areas is there the greatest contrast? Which areas have the least contrast?

L

M

N

O

P

_____

_____

_____

V. Complete These Statements

1. At present, most dental x-ray machines operate in the kVp range of _____.

2. The size of the focal area at the anode in the dental x-ray machine influences greatly the _____ of the image.

3. The two types of related densities that are factors in image formation are the _____ and _____ densities.

4. The milliampere range for an intraoral x-ray machine is _____.

5. Image _____ is the visual quality of a radiograph that depends on definition or sharpness.

6. Using an aluminum step wedge, large gray areas occur when using a _____ -kVp setting as compared with a 65-kVp setting.

7. The difference in the degree of blackness between adjacent areas on a radiograph is the _____.

8. Two advantages of the 16-inch FFD over the 8-inch FFD are _____ and _____.

9. In a periapical radiograph, the milliamperage required for an exposure to produce an acceptable radiograph is determined mainly by the _____.

10. Many in the field of dental radiography believe that the human eye can detect changes better in the _____ -kVp to _____ -kVp range.

11. The main disadvantage of the bisecting technique for periapical radiography is _____.

12. The total energy in the x-ray beam in a specific area and at a given time is called the _____.

13. The actual focal area size is _____ than the effective focal area size in a dental x-ray tube.

14. The limiting factor on how small the focal area can be in the dental x-ray tube is the _____.

15. _____ is the term that describes the area of sharpness in an acceptable radiograph.

VI. Multiple Choice

Select the best answer.

1. A 16-inch cylinder is used in the paralleling technique to
    a. reduce secondary radiation
    b. avoid magnification of the image
    c. avoid distortion of the image
    d. avoid superimposition of anatomic structures
    e. facilitate correct vertical angulation of the position-indicating device (PID)

2. As the distance between the end of the PID and the film increases, the
    a. intensity of the x-ray beam decreases
    b. possibility of film fogging decreases
    c. density of the film image increases
    d. possibility of collimator cutoff decreases
    e. sharpness of the film is affected

3. Image sharpness on a radiograph is increased by
    a. using a large focal spot size
    b. using a small focal spot size
    c. increasing OFD
    d. decreasing target skin distance
    e. increasing exposure time

4. You have decided to switch the PID in your office, replacing the 8-inch cylinder with a 16-inch cylinder. Using D-speed film the milliamperage will remain the same, as will the kilovolt peak. The old exposure for lower premolars was 12 impulses; the new exposure to obtain films of equal density will be
    a. 40 impulses
    b. 30 impulses
    c. 20 impulses
    d. 1 second
    e. 48 impulses

5. As stated in the previous question, after changing to a 16-inch PID you decide to change from D- to E-speed film. The new exposure at the same milliamperage and kilovolt peak for the lower premolar will be
    a. 80 impulses
    b. 24 impulses
    c. 10 impulses
    d. 1 second
    e. 30 impulses

6. The most likely cause for a film with very poor definition is
    a. a large focal area
    b. a very short FFD
    c. patient movement
    d. use of the bisecting technique
    e. use of the paralleling technique

7. A radiograph that has many dark and light areas but few gray areas is said to have
    a. high density
    b. low density
    c. high contrast
    d. low contrast
    e. none of the above

8. To increase contrast, the operator should decrease
    a. exposure time
    b. milliamperage
    c. OFD
    d. film speed
    e. kilovolt peak

9. Use of a kilovolt peak between 45 and 65 produces
    a. scatter radiation
    b. fogging
    c. a blurred image
    d. an underexposed film
    e. none of the above

10. The difference in degrees of blackness on a radiograph is called
    a. density
    b. tone
    c. contrast
    d. fogging
    e. shades

11. A long FFD is desirable because
    a. more radiation is absorbed by the tissues
    b. the resulting radiation is more penetrating
    c. more soft radiation strikes the object
    d. the central rays of the primary beam are less divergent
    e. overexposure rarely occurs

12. Radiographs should always be viewed
    a. in a well-lit room
    b. on a viewbox
    c. in the operatory
    d. by holding them up to a ceiling light
    e. using light from a window

13. Which of the following materials is most effective in absorbing x-rays?
    a. gold
    b. composite
    c. enamel
    d. acrylic
    e. dentin

14. If the intensity of a beam of radiation is 12 at a point 12 inches from the target, the intensity of the beam at 24 inches is
    a. 2
    b. 3
    c. 4
    d. 5
    e. 6

15. You have taken a radiograph of a patient. The resulting image is thin (light). The adjustment that should be made for the retake is
    a. reduce the kilovolt peak
    b. reduce the exposure time
    c. increase the milliamperage
    d. reduce the milliamperage
    e. decrease the processing solution temperature

16. If the distance from the source of radiation to the target film is decreased and no other adjustments are made, the resultant radiograph will
    a. be lighter
    b. be darker
    c. be more defined
    d. have an increased penumbra
    e. be unchanged

17. Changing from 75 kVp to 90 kVp will
    a. increase the radiolucency of the resultant radiograph
    b. decrease radiographic density
    c. decrease radiographic contrast
    d. increase radiographic contrast
    e. increase radiographic exposure time

18. Which of the following causes film fog on radiographs?
    a. underexposure
    b. scattered radiation
    c. improper safelighting
    d. light leak in the darkroom
    e. processing solutions that are too cold
       (1) a, b, c,
       (2) a, b, c, d
       (3) a, b, e
       (4) b, c, d
       (5) b, c, d, e
       (6) c, d, e

19. If the PID is 2 inches away from the patient's skin instead of almost touching, the resulting radiograph will be
    a. underexposed
    b. overexposed
    c. overpenetrated
    d. foreshortened
    e. underpenetrated

20. The criteria for an acceptable radiograph include
    a. proper definition
    b. proper detail
    c. sharpness
    d. desirable contrast
    e. desirable density
    f. all of the above

VII. True/False

Select whether each statement is true (**T**) or false (**F**). Circle the correct answer.

1. The two types of related densities that are factors in image formation are the object density and the film density. **T/F**
2. Low-contrast films appear mainly black and white with very few gray tones. **T/F**
3. The smaller the focal area at the anode is, the better the image detail will be. **T/F**
4. The most common focal film distances (FFDs) used in dentistry are 8, 12, and 20 inches. **T/F**
5. Image detail is not affected by movement. **T/F**

Chapter

4

Image Receptors

Educational Objectives

After reading Chapter 4 of the textbook and completing this exercise, the student will
1. Know and understand the imaging systems available in dental radiography today.
2. Be able to apply this knowledge to clinical situations that call for the use of intraoral panoramic or extraoral projections, as well as their processing and duplication.

I. Definitions

Define/explain the following terms.

1. ANSI film rating _____

   _____

2. Characteristic curve _____

   _____

3. Cassette _____

   _____

4. Double emulsion _____

   _____

5. Double-film packet _____

   _____

6. Extraoral projection _____

   _____

7. Film base _____

   _____

8. Film contrast _____

   _____

9. Film duplication _____

   _____

10. Film emulsion _____

_____

11. Film reversal _____

_____

12. Film sensitivity _____

_____

13. Film-screen system _____

_____

14. Fluorescence _____

_____

15. Fog _____

_____

16. Intensifying screen _____

_____

17. Intensifying screen speed _____

_____

18. Orientation dot _____

_____

19. Phosphor _____

_____

20. Rare earth screen _____

_____

II. Comprehension Exercise

1. What determines film speed? What film speed should be used?

2. Why should the dental professional consult the ANSI rating as opposed to the manufacturer's descriptive names when establishing the desired film speed for an exposure?

3. What special precautions must be taken in the darkroom when loading cassettes and processing extraoral film?

4. What are the advantages of using rare earth intensifying screens?

5. Explain the relationship between the size of the silver halide crystals and the detail/definition of the resulting radiograph.

6. What will happen if an intensifying screen is scratched accidentally in the darkroom?

7. Explain the significance of film-screen compatibility.

8. How can the left side of the patient be differentiated from the right on extraoral and panoramic films?

9. How does the use of intensifying screens reduce the radiation needed for radiographs?

10. What is the purpose of the lead foil in the film packet?

11. Name the three main sources of film fog and briefly explain each.

12. Explain the difference between a double-emulsion film and a double-film packet.

13. How would you compare the mAs needed for E-speed film with that needed for D-speed film?

14. Describe the process of radiographic duplication.

15. How would you compare the radiation exposure to the patient using D-speed film with that using E-speed film?

16. What are silver halides? How are they used in dentistry?

17. What determines the speed of an intensifying screen?

18. List three uses for duplicate radiographs in dentistry.

19. Does the emulsion differ on a bitewing from the emulsion on a periapical film? If so, why?

20. Why should intensifying screens be used in extraoral radiography in spite of the loss of definition exhibited on the resultant radiographs?

III. Matching

Match the items in *Column A* with the appropriate items in *Column B*.

Column A

_____ 1. lead foil backing
_____ 2. pediatric film size
_____ 3. film fog
_____ 4. light fog
_____ 5. film density
_____ 6. single emulsion
_____ 7. flexible cassette
_____ 8. occlusal film
_____ 9. intensifying screen
_____ 10. F-speed film
_____ 11. green light
_____ 12. film duplication
_____ 13. orientation dot
_____ 14. film packet
_____ 15. chemical fog

Column B

a. large halide grains
b. gelatin
c. secondary radiation
d. #4
e. panoramic radiography
f. film mounting
g. decreased patient exposure
h. processing solutions
i. third-party payers
j. overall gray appearance
k. film emulsion
l. light leak
m. #0
n. rare earth intensifying screens
o. degree of blackness
p. duplicating film
q. light-tight

IV. Illustrations

1. (Figure 4-1) In this H and D curve explain, which film, *A* or *B*, would give the patient the least amount of radiation exposure.

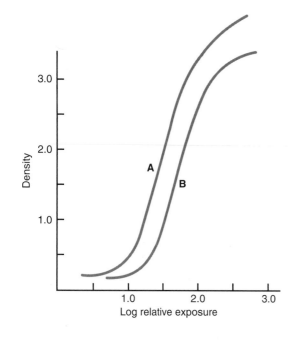

_____

_____

_____

2. (Figure 4-2) Label the film packets with their appropriate film size.

a. _____

b. _____

c. _____

d. _____

e. _____

3. (Figure 4-3) Label (A to F) the components of the intraoral film packet.

a. _____

_____

b. _____

_____

c. _____

_____

d. _____

_____

e. _____

_____

f. _____

_____

4. (Figure 4-4) What is the difference in exposure times between *A* and *B*? Explain.

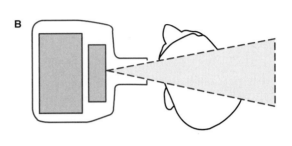

_____

_____

_____

5. (Figure 4-5) What is the relationship between OFD and image magnification as depicted below?

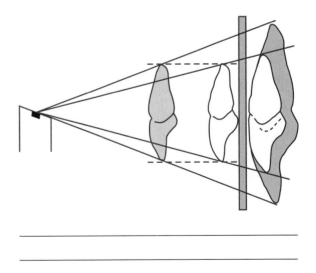

_____

_____

_____

V. Complete These Statements

1. At present the ANSI dental film group that gives the patient the least amount of radiation exposure is _____.

2. The _____ presently used in dentistry are film, electronic sensors, and film-screen combinations.

3. In the early days of dental radiography, the x-ray _____ consisted of glass photographic plates or film cut into pieces and wrapped in black paper or rubber dam.

4. Long bitewing film packets are considered to be size # _____.

5. The plot for dental x-ray film that expresses the relationship between density of the film and the log relative exposure is the _____.

6. Extraoral films are processed in the _____ as intraoral films.

7. The main advantage in using rare earth intensifying screens is _____.

8. F-speed film will reduce radiation exposure by _____ % when compared to D-speed film.

9. When comparing radiographic detail, it can be said that film-screen combinations produce _____ detail when compared to film alone.

10. The component of an x-ray film described as a thin transparent coating that is placed over the emulsion is called the _____.

11. Duplicating film has a _____ emulsion.

12. Duplicating film has the emulsion on the _____ side of the film.

13. Double packets require slightly _____ exposure than single films.

14. It is said that the _____ the silver halide crystals are, the faster the speed of the film.

VI. Multiple Choice

Select the best answer.

1. When comparing ANSI film rated D with ANSI film rated F, one can say that
   a. F film is less sensitive
   b. F film requires more radiation
   c. F film results in more exposure to the patient
   d. F film requires less exposure time
   e. None of the above

2. Rare earth intensifying screens produce
   a. blue light
   b. red light
   c. green light
   d. ultraviolet light
   e. purple light

3. The best way to clean the intensifying screens in extraoral cassettes is with
   a. detergent
   b. disinfectant solution
   c. cold sterilizing solution
   d. soapy water
   e. a wire brush

4. Film fog occurs when all or part of a radiograph is darkened by
   a. an imbalance or exhaustion of processing solutions
   b. a light leak
   c. improper safelighting
   d. scatter radiation
   e. All of the above are potential sources.

5. Which of the following statement is false concerning film duplication?
   a. The films to be duplicated are in close contact with the duplicating film.
   b. The shiny side of the film is the nonemulsion side.
   c. If less film density is needed on the duplicate radiograph, the exposure time is shortened.
   d. The raised portion of the orientation dot faces toward the light source.
   e. The radiographs being duplicated should be removed from their respective mounts.

6. Flexible cassettes are
   a. not used because of cracking of the emulsion
   b. are used in all panoramic units
   c. are used in some panoramic units
   d. are used for lateral oblique projections only
   e. none of the above

7. Intraoral film packets must be
   a. resistant to salivary seepage
   b. flexible
   c. light-tight
   d. easy to open in the darkroom
   e. all of the above

8. To what does the term *film speed* refer?
   a. the developing time needed
   b. sensitivity to x-radiation
   c. half-life
   d. degree of blackness on the exposed radiograph
   e. shelf life

9. The advantage of a film that has emulsion on both sides is that
   a. the film requires less radiation exposure
   b. the image produced is less distorted
   c. the film has less sensitivity to radiation
   d. processing solutions work better
   e. the film is easier to mount

10. Which of the following film sizes is considered to be standard adult film?
    a. size #0
    b. size #1
    c. size #2
    d. size #3
    e. size #4

11. Nonscreen film is routinely used in extraoral radiography.
    a. true
    b. false

12. The intensifying screen that emits blue light and must be used with film that is sensitive to blue light is a
    a. nonlight screen
    b. calcium tungstate screen
    c. rare tungstate screen
    d. rare earth screen
    e. phosphor calcium screen

13. The device that converts x-ray energy into visible light is called a(n)
    a. cassette holder
    b. step-down transformer
    c. intensifying screen
    d. nonscreen film
    e. screen film

14. If the intensifying screens are not in perfect contact with the film, which of the following will occur?
    a. The screen may be damaged.
    b. The film may be damaged.
    c. There will be a light leak.
    d. There will be a loss of image sharpness.
    e. A thin film will result.

15. What is the major advantage in using the fastest speed film and high kilovolt peak?
    a. It increases film density.
    b. It increases film contrast.
    c. It produces a clearer image.
    d. It reduces the radiation exposure to the patient.
    e. It makes film easier and faster to develop.

VII. True/False

Select whether each statement is true (**T**) or false (**F**). Circle the correct answer.

1. The orientation dot on the film packet is useful in mounting. **T/F**
2. The lead foil in the film packet prevents collimator cut-off. **T/F**
3. The use of intensifying screens decreases exposure time. **T/F**
4. Pediatric film is size #3. **T/F**
5. D-speed film is currently recommended for use in dental radiography. **T/F**

Chapter

5

Biologic Effects
of Radiation

Educational Objectives

After reading Chapter 5 of the textbook and completing this exercise, the student will
1. Understand the biologic effects of ionizing radiation on human tissue.
2. Be able to relate these concepts to clinical dental radiology.

I. Definitions

Define/explain the following terms.

1. Acute effects _____

_____

2. ALARA principle _____

_____

3. Background radiation _____

_____

4. Cell recovery _____

_____

5. Chronic effects _____

_____

6. Critical organs _____

_____

7. Dose _____

_____

8. Dose equivalent _____

_____

9. Erythema dose _____

_____

10. Exposure _____

_____

11. Genetic cells _____

_____

12. Indirect effects of radiation _____

_____

13. Latent period _____

_____

14. Primary radiation _____

_____

15. Radiation caries _____

_____

16. Rem _____

_____

17. Risk estimate _____

_____

18. Secondary radiation _____

_____

19. Somatic cells _____

_____

20. Threshold effect _____

_____

II. Comprehension Exercise

1. Explain the difference between radiation exposure and radiation dose.

2. What news events have created public concern of radiation exposure? What can dental professionals do to allay the fears associated with these occurrences?

3. What is the difference between a roentgen, a rad, and a rem?

4. What is the output of an x-ray machine? How is it measured?

5. Explain why the walls of the dental operatory do not become radioactive after continuous exposure to radiation.

6. Explain the difference between a localized dose and a total body dose.

7. What body cells are the most sensitive to ionizing radiation?

8. What is the difference between direct or indirect effects? Which of the two is more prevalent?

9. What is the primary mechanism for tissue change resulting from dental x-ray exposure?

10. Approximately what is the facial exposure from a full-mouth x-ray survey? How is it calculated?

11. How much background radiation does the population at sea level receive each year? What are the major sources of background radiation?

12. How does one handle the dental radiographic needs of a pregnant patient?

13. What are mutations? What can cause mutations in offspring?

14. Name some risks encountered in everyday living that compare with the risks of developing cancer from dental radiation.

15. Explain the risk vs. benefit concept.

16. What is the difference between primary and secondary radiation?

17. What is the erythema dose for facial skin? Is this an important consideration in dental radiology?

18. What does the latent period refer to in dental radiology?

19. What are the units for measuring radiation based on the metric system? How do these units relate to the conventional system?

20. Explain the difference between the acute and chronic effects of radiation.

III. Matching

Match the items in *Column A* with the appropriate items in *Column B*.

Column A

_____ 1. photoelectric effect
_____ 2. rad
_____ 3. total body exposure
_____ 4. ionization
_____ 5. acute effects of radiation
_____ 6. sievert
_____ 7. indirect effects of radiation
_____ 8. attenuation
_____ 9. dose equivalent
_____ 10. leukemia risk
_____ 11. Thompson scatter
_____ 12. roentgen
_____ 13. Compton effect
_____ 14. cell recovery
_____ 15. radiation therapy

Column B

a. free radical formation
b. happens 30% of the time
c. reduced x-ray beam intensity
d. more than 100 rads
e. coherent scatter
f. nuclear accident
g. 100 erg/g
h. cells' repair process
i. low-level radiation
j. radiation caries
k. happens 62% of the time
l. 100 rem
m. qualifying factor
n. free radicals
o. 1 esu/cc of air
p. kilovoltage
q. absorption of x-rays

IV. Illustrations

1. Draw and label a linear nonthreshold dose-response curve.

2. Illustrate the Compton effect of x-ray interaction.

3. Draw a patient's face and illustrate primary and secondary radiation (as found in Chapter 6 of the textbook).

4. Illustrate the difference between localized and total body exposure on a figure of a seated patient.

5. Draw a nonlinear threshold dose-response curve.

V. Complete These Statements

1. The type of interaction between an x-ray photon and a loosely bound orbital electron is characterized by the _____ effect.

2. A pregnant woman in her sixth month can have, if deemed necessary, _____ _____.

3. Radiation from medicine and dentistry accounts for about _____ % of the average annual dose equivalent to the U.S. population.

4. The tissue most sensitive to ionizing radiation is _____.

5. Cellular changes caused by ionizing radiation are not passed on to succeeding generations in _____ tissue.

6. Our objective for the dental radiographic patient is to use the least amount of radiation to obtain _____ _____.

7. The rate at which exposure to ionizing radiation occurs is called the _____.

8. The major component of background radiation at sea level is _____.

9. The objective for occupational radiation exposure is to keep the exposure as close to _____ as possible.

10. The time that elapses between the exposure to ionizing radiation and the appearance of clinical symptoms is called the _____.

11. In considering dental radiology the roentgen, the rad, and the rem are _____.

12. One gray of radiation is equal to _____ rads.

13. An average skin exposure to the patient's face using E-speed film for a full-mouth series is about _____.

14. The two mechanisms for tissue damage resulting from radiation exposure are _____ and _____ formation.

15. An example of an energy wave that will not cause ionization is _____, or _____.

16. An exposure of radiation is measured in _____.

17. The dose-response curve for dental radiation is a _____.

18. An _____ _____ placed in front of a dental x-ray machine's position-indicating (PID) device can indicate how many roentgens the machine is producing per second.

19. The occupational hazard for the pregnant dental professional under proper conditions should be _____.

20. The greatest somatic hazard to patients from dental x-rays is _____.

VI. Multiple Choice

Select the best answer.

1. In taking dental radiographs the greatest dose of radiation to structures in the patient's jaw comes from
   a. the primary beam
   b. leakage from the x-ray machine
   c. scatter from the patient's face
   d. scatter from the PID
   e. secondary radiation

2. Ionization has occurred when
   a. cell death occurs
   b. photons penetrate matter
   c. radiant energy is converted to heat
   d. an electron is displaced from its orbit
   e. none of the above

3. Which form of radiation can cause ionization of atoms?
   a. radar
   b. microwaves
   c. radio waves
   d. visible light
   e. gamma rays

4. The ALARA principle refers to
   a. obtaining informed consent
   b. the disinfection procedures recommended in dental radiography
   c. obtaining diagnostically acceptable radiographs with minimal exposure to radiation
   d. decreasing the processing time for exposed radiographs
   e. none of the above

5. Patient radiation dose is related to which of the following?
   a. length of the exposure
   b. distance from the source
   c. shielding and filtration
   d. time of day
   e. position of the operator
      (1) a, b
      (2) a, b, c
      (3) a, b, c, d
      (4) a, c
      (5) none of the above

6. Which of the following travel at the greatest speed?
   a. x-rays
   b. gamma rays
   c. light
   d. microwaves
   e. they all travel at the same speed

7. X-rays that are most likely to be absorbed by the skin are
   a. those with a short wavelength
   b. aluminum filtered rays
   c. those with long wavelengths
   d. high-energy waves
   e. sonic waves

8. Which of the following statements concerning background radiation is most accurate?
   a. It gives us the maximum recommended dosage for radiation exposure.
   b. It can be avoided if an individual is cautious.
   c. It is found everywhere.
   d. It is only present in dental offices and medical facilities.
   e. None of the above are correct.

9. Arrange the following cells and tissues from most sensitive to least sensitive to ionizing radiation.
   a. nerve
   b. bone
   c. lymphocytes
   d. gastrointestinal tract
      (1) b, a, d, c
      (2) c, a, d, b
      (3) c, b, a, d
      (4) c, d, a, b
      (5) c, d, b, a

10. In recent years the focus of prime concern from the effects of ionizing radiation used in dentistry has centered on
    a. somatic damage to the patient
    b. occupational exposure of dental workers
    c. genetic damage to patients
    d. cancer induction in patients
    e. its contribution to background radiation

11. Under the new metric system for measuring dose (SI), the rem is replaced by the
    a. rad
    b. gray
    c. sievert
    d. becquerel
    e. curie

12. Which of the following types of scatter radiation occurs most often with dental x-rays?
    a. Thompson
    b. Compton
    c. photoelectric
    d. coherent
    e. All of the above occur equally with dental x-rays.

13. The time period between exposure to x-rays and appearance of radiation damage is the
    a. silent period
    b. latent period
    c. waiting period
    d. refractory period
    e. gestation period

14. The Compton effect describes
    a. one type of interaction of x-rays with matter
    b. cell death
    c. cell recovery
    d. cell aberration
    e. cancerous change

15. The ALARA concept means
    a. always lower amperage requirements with age
    b. as low as reasonably achievable
    c. as low as recording allows
    d. as level as reasonably achievable
    e. none of the above

16. An angstrom unit is used to measure
    a. radiation dose
    b. radiation exposure
    c. x-ray wavelength
    d. half-value layer
    e. amperage

17. Which of the following statements are correct?
    a. X-rays can affect all living biologic tissue.
    b. Developing young immature cells are more sensitive to radiation.
    c. In dentistry only the primary beam is of concern for safety.
    d. Changes in adult cells are of short duration and are soon dissipated.
    (1) b, c, d
    (2) a, b, c
    (3) a, c, d, b
    (4) a, b

18. The unit that describes the amount of x-ray exposure in air is the
    a. rad
    b. rem
    c. roentgen
    d. gray
    e. sievert

19. The prime concern for dental personnel taking radiographs under accepted procedures is
    a. primary radiation
    b. secondary radiation
    c. Bremsstrahlung radiation
    d. classical radiation
    e. all of the above

20. Which of the following characteristics of body tissue determines its sensitivity to radiation?
    a. blood flow
    b. iron content
    c. oxyhemoglobin concentration
    d. mitotic rate
    e. water content

VII. True/False

Select whether each statement is true (**T**) or false (**F**). Circle the correct answer.

1. Secondary radiation is the radiation that comes directly from the dental x-ray tube. **T/F**
2. A free radical is an uncharged molecule and is initially very unstable. **T/F**
3. Dose is the amount of ionization in the air produced by x-rays. **T/F**
4. Background radiation can only occur naturally in the environment. **T/F**
5. The reproductive cells are not very radiosensitive. **T/F**

6 Patient Protection

Educational Objectives

After reading Chapter 6 of the textbook and completing this exercise, the student will
1. Understand and be able to practice dental radiography in a safe, efficient manner so that the patient receives the smallest possible dose of radiation as the maximum diagnostic information is acquired.

I. Definitions

Define/explain the following terms.

1. Administrative radiographs _____

_____

2. Collimation _____

_____

3. Film holder _____

_____

4. Filtration _____

_____

5. Head leakage _____

_____

6. Lead apron _____

_____

7. Localizing ring _____

_____

8. Primary radiation _____

_____

9. Radiation history _____

_____

10. Retakes _____

_____

11. Secondary radiation _____

_____

12. Selection criteria _____

_____

13. Thyroid collar _____

_____

14. Tube head drift _____

_____

15. Useful beam _____

_____

II. Comprehension Exercise

1. What is the problem with mechanical timers in dental x-ray machines? Explain.

2. Explain the effect of kilovoltage peak on patient dosage.

3. Why is the use of closed-ended, pointed cones contraindicated in contemporary dentistry?

4. What is the advantage of using F-speed film? Is there a disadvantage? Explain.

5. Why is the paralleling technique preferred over the bisecting technique in regard to patient dosage?

6. What is the relationship between focal-film distance (FFD) and patient dosage?

7. Give some examples of selection criteria for taking radiographs.

8. Why does a technique that employs overexposure with underdevelopment subject the patient to unnecessary radiation? Explain.

9. What is the present status of administrative radiographs?

10. List six major ways to reduce x-ray dose for patients.

III. Matching

Match the items in *Column A* with the appropriate items in *Column B*.

Column A

_____ 1. postoperative radiographs
_____ 2. selection criteria
_____ 3. administrative radiographs
_____ 4. paralleling technique
_____ 5. increased FFD
_____ 6. change from E- to F-speed film
_____ 7. radiation history
_____ 8. mechanical timers
_____ 9. filtration
_____ 10. lead apron

Column B

a. decreased exit dose
b. remove soft wavelengths
c. medical/dental diagnostic and therapeutic radiation
d. root tip retrieval
e. reduce dose by 20%
f. not to be taken
g. inaccurate by ¼ of a second
h. required in many localities
i. inaccurate by a second
j. decreased thyroid dose
k. determines x-rays that are needed
l. 2¾-inch beam diameter

IV. Illustrations

1. Draw the different relationships of the x-ray beam and secondary radiation to the thyroid gland using both the paralleling and bisecting techniques.

2. Illustrate how less tissue volume is exposed using a 16-inch FFD rather than an 8-inch FFD.

V. Complete These Statements

1. In an adult patient not prone to caries and clinically negative, bitewing radiographs should be taken every

   _____ .

2. All new edentulous patients should

   _____

   _____ .

3. Radiographs should always be viewed

   _____ .

4. Taking radiographs to confirm the fit of restorations should be

   _____ .

5. Retaking radiographs because of poor technique results in

   _____ .

6. _____

   _____ is the single most effective factor in reducing radiation exposure to the patient.

7. The thyroid dose in the bisecting method is greater because of

   _____ .

8. The use of F-speed film will

   _____ .

9. Mechanical timers are

   _____ .

10. Kilovoltage of less than 65 should never be used for dental x-rays because

    _____ .

VI. Multiple Choice

Select the best answer.

1. Using an F-speed rather than an E-speed film to produce a radiograph results in
   a. greater patient exposure
   b. less patient exposure
   c. the same exposure time
   d. a longer processing time
   e. a shorter processing time

2. All of the following reduce radiation exposure to the patient except
   a. rectangular collimation
   b. fast-speed film
   c. overexposure with underdevelopment
   d. lead aprons
   e. aluminum filtration

3. Which of the following combinations of dose reduction methods is most effective for reducing radiation for patients?
   a. E-speed film, round collimation
   b. E-speed film, lead apron
   c. D-speed film, rectangular collimation
   d. E-speed film, rectangular collimation
   e. D-speed film, lead apron

4. A dental x-ray machine operating at 75 kVp is required to have a total aluminum filtration of
   a. 2 mm
   b. 2.5 mm
   c. 2 inches
   d. 2.5 inches
   e. 2.75 inches

5. Every radiographic retake represents
   a. an impulse of additional exposure to the patient
   b. a quadrupling of exposure to the patient
   c. an unnecessary doubling of patient exposure
   d. an attempt to improve one's technique without cost to the patient
   e. None of the above are relevant.

6. Which of these position-indicating devices (PIDs) is least effective in minimizing radiation scatter?
   a. lead-lined cylinder
   b. pointed cone
   c. lead-lined rectangle
   d. plastic cylinder
   e. plastic rectangle

7. Radiation history should include all of the following except
   a. medical radiation exposure
   b. dental radiation exposure
   c. therapeutic radiation exposure
   d. background radiation exposure
   e. panoramic radiation exposure

8. Lead aprons should be used
   a. on all patients
   b. to reassure patients
   c. to reduce scatter to the film
   d. only on children
   e. only on pregnant patients

9. All but which of the following are important to minimize patient exposure to radiation?
   a. proper collimation
   b. not utilizing selection criteria to prescribe radiographs
   c. proper filtration
   d. darkroom quality assurance programs
   e. history taking

10. Dental radiographs should be taken
    a. only if there is pain
    b. to train students
    c. for insurance company requests
    d. routinely every 6 months
    e. to aid in diagnosis

11. Which of the following results in the greatest reduction to radiation in the patient?
    a. short developing time
    b. low kilovoltage peak
    c. film with fast emulsion speed
    d. wide primary beam
    e. high milliamperage

12. According to selection criteria
    a. an asymptomatic edentulous patient does not require radiographs
    b. a 14-year-old patient will probably need posterior bitewings
    c. a panoramic exam is needed for a new edentulous patient
    d. very few patients need radiographs at 6-month intervals
    e. All of the above are correct.

13. The maximum diameter of the dental x-ray beam measured at the skin should be no greater than
    a. 2 mm
    b. 2.75 inches
    c. 2 inches
    d. 2.5 inches
    e. 2.75 mm

14. Before prescribing dental radiographs, which of the following are needed?
    a. history of previous radiographs
    b. clinical examination
    c. medical history
    d. dental history
    e. all of the above

15. The most important use of x-rays in dentistry is
    a. patient education
    b. legal protection
    c. diagnosis
    d. pain control
    e. therapy

VII. True/False

Select whether each statement is true (**T**) or false (**F**). Circle the correct answer.

1. The ALARA principle deals with radiation protection of the patient and operator. **T/F**
2. Pregnant patients may have radiographs taken when they are needed. **T/F**
3. The closed-ended pointed PID is recommended for use in dental radiography. **T/F**
4. Administrative radiographs should be strongly discouraged. **T/F**
5. The dose to the thyroid gland is greater in the bisecting angle technique. **T/F**

Operator Protection

Educational Objectives

After reading Chapter 7 of the textbook and completing this exercise, the student will
1. Understand and feel comfortable working with ionizing radiation.

I. Definitions

Define/explain the following terms.

1. Exposure technique _____

_____

2. Film badge _____

_____

3. Ionizing chamber _____

_____

4. Maximum permissible dose (MPD) _____

_____

5. Monitoring device _____

_____

6. Pocket dosimeter _____

_____

7. Protective barrier _____

_____

8. Radiation monitoring _____

_____

9. Radiation survey _____

_____

10. W × U × T _____

_____

II. Comprehension Exercise

1. What does the acronym "CRESO" represent, and how does it apply to operator protection?

2. Where should the operator be positioned when taking radiographs?

3. Explain the significance of the present levels of the MPD.

4. What are the sources of potential radiation exposure to the radiographer?

5. What constitutes adequate shielding in the dental office? Are lead-lined walls always necessary?

6. What is the equation for determining the accumulated lifetime dose for a dental radiographer? What would it be for a 35-year-old?

7. What are the advantages of personnel wearing film badges over a radiation survey?

8. What should the operator "not do" in order to avoid primary beam exposure during a dental radiographic procedure?

9. Can dental workers continue to take radiographs during pregnancy? Explain.

10. List the ways the operator's occupational dose can be kept to zero.

III. Matching

Match the items in *Column A* with the appropriate items in *Column B*.

Column A

_____ 1. occupational MPD
_____ 2. nonoccupational MPD
_____ 3. maximum scatter
_____ 4. film badge
_____ 5. monitoring device
_____ 6. CRESO
_____ 7. lead-lined walls
_____ 8. 6 feet away
_____ 9. minimum scatter
_____ 10. barrier

Column B

a. right angles to the x-ray beam
b. 5000 mrem
c. not always necessary
d. 50 rem/year
e. radiation shielding
f. radiation survey
g. personal radiation exposure
h. filtration
i. 500 mrem
j. proper operator position
k. lead apron
l. behind the patient
m. pocket dosimeter

IV. Illustrations

1. Draw a diagram of a dental operatory and indicate where the operator should stand when making a radiographic exposure.

2. Draw a diagram identifying the areas of minimum and maximum scatter during dental x-ray exposure.

V. Complete These Statements

1. Three factors used in calculating the type of barrier needed in a dental office are _____, _____, and _____.

2. The two methods that can alert dental personnel to the amount of occupational exposure they are receiving are through a _____ and by wearing a _____.

3. A full-mouth series is equivalent to about _____ days of background radiation exposure.

4. The MPD for occupational exposure to ionizing radiation will be _____ _____.

5. If a pregnant operator follows proper procedure, there is _____ _____ to the fetus.

6. _____ construction, if of proper thickness, is sufficient for proper radiation shielding.

7. A film badge reading of 400 mR for a 4-week period _____ _____.

8. If one is positioned 6 feet from the head of the x-ray machine during an exposure, then _____.

9. Under no circumstance should the dental professional _____.

10. Operators should not wear their film badges _____ their offices.

VI. Multiple Choice

Select the best answer.

1. At present the recommended MPD for nonoccupationally exposed individuals is
   a. 500 mrem/year
   b. 5 mrem/year
   c. 5 rem/year
   d. 5000 mrem/year
   e. 0.5 mrem/year

2. The occupational radiation dose will be kept to zero if _____
   a. careful technique is employed
   b. the office is well designed
   c. the office is well monitored
   d. the office is well equipped
   e. All of the above are correct.

3. The MPD is best defined as
   a. the maximum dose of radiation a patient should receive from dental exposures
   b. the permissible amount of radiation that causes cancer in human populations
   c. the maximum dose of ionizing radiation that is not expected to cause injury
   d. the amount of radiation that kills 50% of a population in 30 days
   e. none of the above

4. By having the operator stand 6 feet rather than 3 feet from a radiation source, the resultant exposure is decreased by a factor of
   a. 2
   b. 4
   c. 6
   d. 8
   e. 10

5. The International Commission on Radiation Protection (ICRP) has recommended that the yearly MPD for operators not exceed
   a. 5 mrem
   b. 500 mrem
   c. 50 mrem
   d. 5000 mrem
   e. 5.5 mrem

6. Workload determination for dental x-ray machine room barriers requires knowledge of
   a. milliamperage
   b. exposure time per film
   c. number of exposures per week
   d. adjacent room location
   e. experience of operator
      (1) a, d, e
      (2) a, b, c
      (3) a, b, c, d
      (4) c, d, e
      (5) a, c, d, e

7. What can be used to check the reliability of the x-ray machine and protective barriers?
   a. film badge
   b. ionizing chamber
   c. pocket dosimeter
   d. coin test
   e. a, b, and c only

8. Which of the following is true regarding film badges?
   a. They should be worn when dental personnel have radiographs as a patient.
   b. Film badges can be shared by employees.
   c. Film badges can be worn outside the office.
   d. Film badges should be worn so as not to be blocked by pens or jewelry.
   e. None of the above is correct.

9. Which of the following, if sufficient, could provide adequate shielding?
   a. lead-lined walls
   b. dry wall construction
   c. cinder block walls
   d. concrete walls
   e. All of the above could be adequate.

10. What is the main source of radiation exposure to the operator?
   a. primary radiation
   b. scatter radiation
   c. background radiation
   d. tertiary radiation
   e. none of the above

VII. True/False

Select whether each statement is true (**T**) or false (**F**). Circle the correct answer.

1. Operators of dental x-ray machines should be 4 feet away from the source of radiation. **T/F**
2. Lead-lined walls in a dental operatory are not mandatory. **T/F**
3. Film badges are always required in a dental office. **T/F**
4. The MPD for occupationally exposed individuals in the dental office per week is 100 mrem. **T/F**
5. Selection criteria are guidelines established to mandate barrier protection in the operatory. **T/F**

Chapter

8

Film Processing: The Darkroom

Educational Objectives

After reading Chapter 8 of the textbook and completing this exercise, the student will

1. Understand the theory of film processing and how to operate and maintain a darkroom.
2. Be able to process radiographs and identify and correct errors made in the darkroom.

I. Definitions

Define/explain the following terms.

1. Archival life _____
   _____

2. Automatic processing _____
   _____

3. Clear film _____
   _____

4. Coin test _____
   _____

5. Darkroom _____
   _____

6. Daylight loader _____
   _____

7. Developer cutoff _____
   _____

8. Film fog _____
   _____

9. Film hangers _____
   _____

10. Latent image _____

_____

11. Manual processing _____

_____

12. Rapid processing _____

_____

13. Reference film _____

_____

14. Replenisher solutions _____

_____

15. Safelight_____

_____

16. Sight developing _____

_____

17. Silver retrieval _____

_____

18. Thermostatic valve _____

_____

19. Time-temperature processing _____

_____

20. Wet reading _____

_____

II. Comprehension Exercise

1. List, describe, and state the purpose of each step involved in the manual processing of dental x-ray film.

2. What is the primary precaution that should be taken when processing extraoral radiographs? Why?

3. How do you test for safelight reliability?

4. Why is the time-temperature technique the best method for processing radiographs?

5. List and explain the three types of wastes that can be generated as a result of dental radiography.

6. Is sight developing an acceptable technique? Why or why not?

7. Why is it not acceptable to underdevelop a film to compensate for overexposure of the same film?

8. What is the major advantage of automatic processing? Explain.

9. List the chemicals that make up the developer and fixer solutions and identify the function of each.

10. What are the clinical indications for rapid processing? What are the disadvantages?

11. List two ways to check the strength of the processing solutions as a component of the quality assurance program and explain each method.

12. When must safelight conditions be maintained in the darkroom?

13. What are the responsibilities of the dental support team in the darkroom?

14. Define reticulation and describe the cause and remedy related to this processing error.

15. Distinguish between the appearance of collimator cutoff and developer cutoff on the finished radiograph.

16. Can one distinguish between an overexposed film and an overdeveloped film? How?

17. What can cause a clear film?

18. Discuss the importance of a quality assurance program in the darkroom.

19. When should processing solutions be changed?

20. What causes white lines on a finished radiograph? Black lines?

21. What will happen if film is left in the fixer solution over a weekend?

22. What should you do if succeeding panoramic films appear increasingly light?

23. Why is it important to maintain the levels of the processing solutions? How often should the levels be checked? What should be done to maintain the adequate levels?

24. What are the factors that should be considered when determining the space needed for a darkroom?

25. Name the five different light sources in a well-designed darkroom and provide the purpose for each.

III. Matching

Match the items in *Column A* with the appropriate items in *Column B*.

Column A

_____ 1. coin test
_____ 2. lost films in tank
_____ 3. underdeveloped film
_____ 4. static marks
_____ 5. excessive fixing
_____ 6. overdeveloped film
_____ 7. energized silver bromide
_____ 8. radiolucent bands on film
_____ 9. sodium carbonate
_____ 10. thermometer
_____ 11. air bubbles
_____ 12. unaffected silver bromide
_____ 13. energized silver
_____ 14. overlapped films
_____ 15. change solutions

Column B

a. latent image
b. agitate film hangers
c. dense image
d. 2 to 3 weeks
e. softens gelatin
f. films fed too quickly
g. hardens gelatin crystals
h. clear films
i. thin image
j. safelight check
k. dirty rollers
l. "wet elbow"
m. fixer precipitated
n. forcefully open packet
o. developer
p. reticulation
q. kept in the developer

IV. Illustrations

1. (Figure 8-1) What stages of the developing process are seen diagrammatically in this figure (1, 2, 3 and 4)?

Metallic filling
Pulp
Caries
Dentin
Enamel
Air

1

2

3

4

1. _____

2. _____

3. _____

4. _____

2. (Figure 8-2) List two possible causes for the film fog seen in this figure.

_____

_____

_____

3. (Figure 8-3) Identify the error seen in this figure.

_____

_____

_____

4. (Figure 8-4) Name three possible causes that could produce a film like that seen in this figure.

_____

_____

_____

6. (Figure 8-6) What error results in the artifacts seen in this figure?

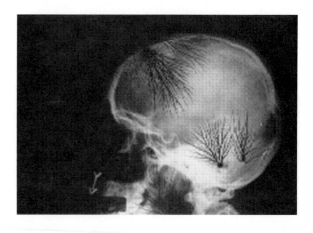

_____

_____

_____

5. (Figure 8-5) What could cause the error seen in this figure?

_____

_____

_____

7. (Figure 8-7) What error was made in automatic processing to result in this figure?

_____

_____

_____

8. (Figure 8-8) What error produces the film seen in this figure?

_____

_____

_____

9. (Figure 8-9) What error can produce a radiograph such as the one in this figure?

_____

_____

_____

10. (Figure 8-10) Interpret the result of the safelight (coin) test shown in this figure.

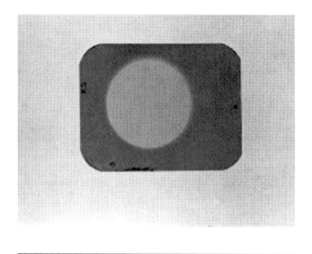

_____

_____

_____

V. Complete These Statements

1. The temperature of the processing chemicals is maintained by

   _____

   _____.

2. If the developer solution contaminates the fixer solution, the operator should

   _____.

3. Two types of light used in the darkroom are _____ and

   _____.

4. Two advantages of automatic processors are _____ and

   _____.

5. A latent image is invisible until the film is

   _____.

6. The easiest way to check a darkroom for light leaks is to

   _____

   _____.

7. At minimum, developer and fixer levels should be checked _____.

8. A manually processed radiograph should be washed for _____ just before drying.

9. The thermometer in a darkroom is always kept in the _____ solution.

10. The levels of the processing chemicals should be maintained by adding _____.

11. Expended fixer solution should be disposed of by _____.

12. To determine whether a safelight is "safe," one should _____.

13. X-ray processing solutions should be stored in a _____, _____ area.

14. For complete fixation, the films should be left in the solution for approximately _____ the developing time.

15. Panoramic films are processed in _____ as intraoral films.

VI. Multiple Choice

1. Each successive full-mouth survey appears lighter than the one before. Which of the following corrections should be made?
   a. Increase the mA setting.
   b. Increase the kVp setting.
   c. Change the intensifying screens.
   d. Change the developer solution.
   e. Decrease the temperature of the developer solution.

2. A major difference between automatic and manual processing of radiographs is that automatic processing
   a. is more expensive
   b. provides better quality films
   c. requires special solutions at higher temperatures
   d. doesn't allow for processing errors
   e. allows for more latitude in exposure techniques

3. In developing radiographs, the fixer acts to
   a. prevent film fog and soften the emulsion
   b. remove exposed silver halide and soften the emulsion
   c. remove exposed silver halide and shrink and harden the emulsion
   d. remove unexposed and undeveloped silver halide from the film and harden the emulsion
   e. prevent reticulation and harden the emulsion

4. If the temperature of the processing solutions is slightly above normal, radiographs of desired density may be best obtained by
   a. increasing the fixing time
   b. decreasing the fixing time
   c. increasing the developing time
   d. decreasing the developing time
   e. increasing the exposure time

5. A latent image is
   a. found only on E-speed film
   b. caused only by scattered radiation
   c. prevented by the lead foil in the film packet
   d. invisible until the film is processed
   e. none of the above

6. An exposed radiograph should remain in the fixer in order to attain archival life for
   a. as long as it remains in the developer
   b. until the film clears
   c. twice the developing time
   d. a minimum of 1 hour
   e. 5 minutes at 70°F

7. Which of the following causes dark spots during film development?
   a. film contamination with fixer before processing
   b. film contamination with developer before processing
   c. developing solution that is too warm
   d. overdevelopment of the exposed film
   e. none of the above

8. The effect of safelight illumination in the darkroom does not depend on which of the following?
   a. size of the darkroom
   b. type of film used
   c. wattage of the bulb
   d. type of filter used
   e. distance of the safelight from the work surface

9. A radiograph is clear after processing. This could result from any of the following *except*
   a. unexposed film
   b. excessive washing
   c. prolonged fixing
   d. exposure to white light
   e. the x-ray machine was not turned on

10. In treating an emergency patient you remove the radiograph from the fixer bath after 3 minutes and wash it. It is diagnostic. After treatment the film is dried and put in the patient's chart.
    a. This is proper procedure.
    b. This is acceptable procedure.
    c. The film will turn yellowish-brown in a few weeks.
    d. The film should have been returned to the water bath overnight.
    e. None of the above is true.

11. The operator observes that a portion of the processed panoramic radiograph is completely black. What is the most likely cause?
    a. excessive exposure time
    b. exposure to white light
    c. exposure to a light leak
    d. temperature of the developer was too high
    e. patient movement occurred during exposure

12. In the time-temperature method of processing dental radiographs, the thermometer is
    a. not used
    b. kept in the fixer bath
    c. kept in the water bath
    d. kept in the developer bath
    e. not read for the first series processed

13. Which is the correct order for manually processing radiographs?
    a. rinse, develop, fix
    b. develop, fix, wash, dry
    c. develop, rinse, fix, wash, dry
    d. fix, rinse, develop, wash, dry
    e. None of the above is correct.

14. Even though proper exposure techniques were employed, radiographs emerging from an automatic processor exhibit chalky smudges. What is the most likely cause?
    a. improper safelighting
    b. use of outdated film
    c. premature contact with the developer solution
    d. premature contact with the fixer solution
    e. dirty processor rollers

15. Manufacturers recommend that radiographic developing solutions be covered to prevent
    a. evaporation of the solutions
    b. an increase in the strength of the solutions
    c. emission of an oxidizing agent
    d. dilution of the solutions
    e. both a and c are acceptable answers

16. The coin test of a safelight in the darkroom shows a clear outline of the coin. What does this mean?
    a. The developer is exhausted.
    b. The safelight is adequate.
    c. The fixer solution is weak.
    d. The safelight is faulty.
    e. There was inadequate fixation.

17. If films are fed into the automatic processor too rapidly, what can happen?
    a. Films will stick together.
    b. Films will be cracked.
    c. Static electricity will be generated.
    d. Radiographs will be lighter than normal.
    e. Radiographs will be darker than normal.

18. A step-wedge control device would be primarily used
    a. to test the safelight in the darkroom
    b. to evaluate the amount of radiation exposure
    c. to wedge steps of lead into the dental walls to act as a barrier to radiation
    d. for quality assurance of processing solutions
    e. to compare the dental films of one patient to another

19. Which of the following conditions will result in a radiograph that is too light?
    a. The darkroom door is left opened during developing.
    b. Processing solutions are too warm.
    c. The safelight is inadequate.
    d. The automatic processor has a daylight loader.
    e. The developing solution is too weak.

20. Which of the following does not cause film fog in developed radiographs?
    a. underexposure
    b. scatter radiation
    c. improper safelighting
    d. a light leak in the darkroom
    e. processing solutions that are too warm

21. After developing a complete radiographic series, the operator notices that the films on the bottom of the rack are of a different density than those at the top of the rack and concludes that
    a. the developing solution was contaminated
    b. the thermometer is faulty
    c. the fixer solution was reaching exhaustion
    d. the solutions were not stirred
    e. the developing solution was too cold

22. Your last patient before the weekend is a new patient on whom you take a full-mouth series of radiographs. If you process the films that evening,
    a. the films can be left in the water bath
    b. the films can be left in the fixer
    c. the films have to be processed immediately to preserve the latent image
    d. the films can be left in the developer
    e. the films must be processed completely and left to dry

23. One indication for "rapid processing" would be
    a. detection of caries
    b. periodontal bone evaluation
    c. confirming an endodontic measurement
    d. evaluating periapical changes
    e. none of the above

24. The action of the fixer on unenergized silver bromide crystals in the emulsion is to
    a. precipitate them as free silver
    b. fix them to the film base
    c. incorporate them into the hardened gelatin
    d. remove them from the film
    e. reuse them

25. Processing solutions should be changed, depending on usage, about
    a. every week
    b. every day
    c. every month
    d. every 2 to 3 weeks
    e. every 6 months

VII. True/False

Select whether each statement is true (**T**) or false (**F**). Circle the correct answer.

1. Automatic processing is never recommended over manual processing. **T/F**
2. When processing solutions are at a low level, water should be added. **T/F**
3. Expended fixing solutions should be poured down the drain. **T/F**
4. Sight development is a scientifically acceptable procedure of processing. **T/F**
5. The coin test is used to test the level of solutions in the processing tanks. **T/F**

Chapter

9

Infection Control in Dental Practice

Educational Objectives

After reading Chapter 9 of the textbook and completing this exercise, the student will
1. Be able to take and process all radiographs, adhering to and understanding the accepted infection control policy.
2. Be able to prepare and break down a dental operatory after completing patient radiographs.
3. Feel comfortable and assured in treating a patient with an infectious disease by following infection control protocol.

I. Definitions

Define/explain the following terms.

1. AIDS _____

_____

2. Antibiotic prophylaxis _____

_____

3. CDC _____

_____

4. Cold sterilization _____

_____

5. Contamination _____

_____

6. Critical instruments _____

_____

7. Cross-contamination _____

_____

8. Disinfection _____

_____

9. Immunization _____

_____

10. Infection control barriers _____

_____

11. OSHA _____

_____

12. Parental exposure _____

_____

13. Pathogen _____

_____

14. Sterilization _____

_____

15. Universal precautions _____

_____

II. Comprehension Exercise

1. In dental radiography what are the main vectors for cross-contamination?

2. What is the significance of taking a comprehensive medical history on a patient before dental treatment?

3. What are the required barriers that dental personnel must wear while performing radiographic procedures?

Chapter 9: Infection Control in Dental Practice **79**

Copyright © 2011, 2005, 2001, 1996 by Mosby, Inc., an affiliate of Elsevier Inc.

4. What are some of the barriers that can be used for equipment in the operatory when performing radiography?

5. Why is saliva considered to be a possible transmission route for human immunodeficiency virus (HIV) even though transmission via this route has not been documented to date?

6. What is the difference between sterilization and disinfection? How is each used in dental radiology?

7. For which diseases should dental personnel receive immunizations?

8. Describe the use of the processing solutions used in the darkroom in terms of the disinfection and sterilization of the film.

9. What are the infection control requirements concerning protective clothing in dentistry?

10. What are the cross-contamination hazards with the use of a daylight loader?

11. List the infection control procedures that operators should follow before, during, and after the taking of dental radiographs.

12. What is the general consensus regarding antibiotic prophylaxis and dental radiographic procedures?

13. Describe three ways to handle contaminated film packets to avoid contaminating the film.

14. What is a barrier film packet? Describe its use.

15. What type of infection control procedures is necessary when using an automatic processor with a daylight loader? Without a daylight loader?

16. What is "cold sterilization"? Is it appropriate for use in dental radiography?

17. What is the problem in using disinfecting solutions instead of barriers with the dental x-ray machine?

18. Discuss the disadvantages of using gloves, mask, and eyewear when performing dental radiographic procedures.

19. What are the infection control procedures needed when taking a panoramic radiograph?

20. Explain the following statement and its clinical significance: "All pathogens are microorganisms, but not all microorganisms are pathogens."

III. Matching

Match the items in *Column A* with the appropriate items in *Column B*.

Column A

_____ 1. AIDS
_____ 2. immunization
_____ 3. pathogen
_____ 4. barriers
_____ 5. disinfecting solution
_____ 6. sterilization
_____ 7. cold sterilization
_____ 8. antiseptic agent
_____ 9. barrier envelope
_____ 10. saliva
_____ 11. previous endocarditis
_____ 12. semicritical instrument
_____ 13. critical instrument
_____ 14. occupational exposure
_____ 15. film packet

Column B

a. film
b. main vector
c. antibiotic prophylaxis
d. no vaccine
e. hepatitis B
f. contaminant
g. protects film
h. patient's chart
i. soap
j. periodontal probe
k. gloves, mask, eyewear, gowns
l. steam autoclave
m. iodophor
n. film-holding device
o. not recommended
p. causes disease

IV. Illustrations

Identify the errors illustrated in Figures 9-1 through 9-5.

1. (Figure 9-1)

_____

_____

_____

2. (Figure 9-2)

_____

_____

_____

3. (Figure 9-3)

_____

_____

_____

4. (Figure 9-4)

_____
_____
_____

5. (Figure 9-5)

_____
_____
_____

V. Complete These Statements

1. Even before the advent of AIDS, _____ and _____ had always been a risk for dental professionals.

2. _____ is the most common and easily recognized transmission route of HIV, HBV, and HCV.

3. AIDS and HIV are abbreviations for _____ and _____.

4. When taking intraoral radiographs, _____, _____, _____, and _____ should be worn at all times.

5. All dental professionals should be immunized for _____.

6. The most common methods of sterilization used in the dental office are _____ _____ and the use of the _____.

7. Infection control procedures require that every patient be treated _____.

8. Three vehicles for the transmission of pathogens on intraoral film holders are _____, _____, and _____.

9. Other than the operator's hands, the _____ is considered to be the main source of cross-contamination in dental radiography.

10. Anything that the operator touches after removing the exposed film packet from the patient's mouth must be considered _____.

11. All working surfaces and the dental x-ray unit should be _____ before radiographs are taken.

12. Cold sterilization is _____ an acceptable method for use for intraoral film-holding devices.

13. _____ can be contaminated by blood and therefore poses a potential for transmission of infectious organisms.

14. Film packets are considered _____ after they are removed from the patient's mouth.

15. The developing and fixing solutions used in the darkroom have not been shown to act as _____ agents.

VI. Multiple Choice

Select the best answer.

1. In dental radiography, which of the following infection control procedures is used?
   a. sterilization
   b. disinfection
   c. antiseptic agents
   d. instant hand sanitizer
   e. all of the above

2. If the barrier envelope is not used
   a. operators could open the packet without gloves.
   b. operators should remove the films while wearing the same gloves used for exposure.
   c. operators should take care not to touch the films as they are dropped onto a clean surface
   d. operators could touch anything on the way to the darkroom with the previously contaminated gloves.
   e. none of the above

3. Daylight loaders are not recommended for infection control because of
   a. strength of the processing solutions
   b. time delay
   c. possibility of cross-contamination within the confined area of the loader
   d. light leaks
   e. none of the above

4. Infection control procedures should be followed for
   a. patients known to have AIDS
   b. patients who are HIV positive
   c. patients with an alternative lifestyle
   d. all patients
   e. non-compliant patients

5. Any contaminated film that is processed
   a. emerges from the processor sterilized
   b. emerges from the processor disinfected
   c. emerges from the processor decontaminated
   d. emerges from the processor still contaminated
   e. none of the above

6. With the use of a barrier envelope
   a. no other precautions are necessary
   b. gloves are not necessary after the film has been removed from the packs
   c. processing is less difficult
   d. processing is more difficult
   e. an increased exposure time is needed

7. Developer and fixer solutions
   a. do not act as sterilizing agents
   b. are antiseptic
   c. act as sterilizing agents
   d. destroy all viruses
   e. none of the above

8. Autoclaving a contaminated exposed film packet
   a. is not recommended because it takes too long
   b. does not sterilize the packet
   c. destroys the image
   d. refines the image
   e. none of the above

9. Every patient should have a current medical history that
   a. is obtained through a questionnaire
   b. is obtained through direct questioning
   c. alerts the dental team to the presence or history of infectious disease
   d. All of the above are valid statements.
   e. None of the above are valid statements.

10. Immersing the contaminated exposed film packet in a disinfecting solution
    a. destroys the image
    b. is recommended
    c. takes too long
    d. none of the above
    e. all of the above

11. Using disinfecting solutions on the dental x-ray unit is not recommended because
    a. of the cost involved
    b. of the time involved
    c. it is not effective
    d. the solution may seep into the electrical connections
    e. none of the above

12. Microorganisms can remain viable on radiographic equipment for at least
    a. 72 hours
    b. 48 hours
    c. 10 hours
    d. 24 hours
    e. none of the above

13. When taking bitewings on a patient with a negative medical history
    a. gloves and eyewear should be used
    b. just gloves are necessary
    c. gloves, eyeglasses, protective clothing, and masks should be worn
    d. eyeglasses are not necessary
    e. none of the above

14. When taking a full-mouth series of radiographs
    a. the exposure switch should be covered with plastic
    b. the PID need not be covered if gloves are worn
    c. a film dispenser should not be used
    d. unexposed film should be kept in the room
    e. none of the above

15. The infection control procedure for daylight loaders includes
    a. preparing the interior of the daylight loader before processing
    b. placing clean hands through the sleeve baffles
    c. opening packets with clean gloves
    d. All of the above are true statements.
    e. None of the above are true statements.

VII. True/False

Select whether each statement is true (**T**) or false (**F**). Circle the correct answer.

1. An antiseptic is a substance that inhibits the growth of bacteria. **T/F**
2. Sterilization is the process of destroying disease-causing microorganisms by physical or chemical means. **T/F**
3. Every patient should not be treated in the same manner such as with universal precautions. **T/F**
4. The processing procedure for films with and without barrier envelopes is exactly the same. **T/F**
5. In panoramic radiography more areas are contaminated by the patient's saliva. **T/F**

Intraoral Technique: The Paralleling Method

Copyright © 2011, 2005, 2001, 1996 by Mosby, Inc., an affiliate of Elsevier Inc.

Educational Objectives

After reading Chapter 10 of the textbook and completing this exercise, the student will

1. Understand the geometry of the x-ray beam direction and film placement.
2. Be able to apply these principles to take a full-mouth survey of radiographs for dentulous and edentulous adult or pediatric patients.
3. Recognize unacceptable radiographs and their causes and know how to correct the errors.

I. Definitions

Define/explain the following terms.

1. Bitewing radiograph _____

_____

2. Blurred image _____

_____

3. Collimator cutoff _____

_____

4. Dimensional accuracy _____

_____

5. Double exposure _____

_____

6. Exposure time _____

_____

7. Film reversal _____

_____

8. Full-mouth survey (series) _____

_____

9. Horizontal angulation _____

_____

10. Localizing ring _____

_____

11. Overexposure _____

_____

12. Overlapping _____

_____

13. Paralleling method _____

_____

14. Pediatric full-mouth survey (series) _____

_____

15. Periapical radiograph _____

_____

16. Point of entry _____

_____

17. Sagittal plane orientation _____

_____

18. Underexposure _____

_____

19. Vertical angulation _____

_____

20. Vertical bitewing radiograph _____

_____

II. Comprehension Exercise

1. Explain why it is necessary in a full-mouth series to take radiographs of edentulous areas.

2. What would be the indication for use of vertical bitewing projections?

3. Describe what an elongated radiograph looks like.

4. What is the importance of correct horizontal angulation?

5. List/explain two helpful hints for placement of the mandibular anterior projection.

6. What are the two main principles of the paralleling method?

7. What is the purpose of using a localizing ring?

8. Describe the film position for a maxillary molar projection.

9. How does the consequence of inadequate closure appear on a radiograph?

10. Describe what a foreshortened radiograph would look like.

11. Why does one remove nonfixed appliances from the patient's mouth when taking radiographs?

12. What can cause a blurred image?

13. Name three chairside technique errors that will result in a thin (light) film.

14. How does a cracked emulsion due to overbending the film packet appear on the radiograph?

15. List the criteria that determine whether a radiograph is considered diagnostic.

16. Why is there no superimposition of the zygomatic arch on maxillary molars in the paralleling technique?

17. Can the paralleling method be used with an 8-inch focal-film distance (FFD)? Explain.

18. What determines how many films there will be in a pediatric full-mouth survey?

19. List/describe one way to avoid double-exposed projections.

20. What action would you take before using the bisecting angle technique if parallel positioning of the film is difficult on a pediatric patient?

III. Matching

Match the items in *Column A* with the appropriate items in *Column B*.

Column A

_____ 1. proximal surface overlap
_____ 2. collimator cutoff
_____ 3. dense film
_____ 4. "herringbone" effect
_____ 5. thin image (light)
_____ 6. localizing ring
_____ 7. elongation
_____ 8. bitewing projection
_____ 9. residual pathology
_____ 10. loss of definition
_____ 11. bisecting angle technique
_____ 12. 16-inch PID
_____ 13. inadequate vertical angulation
_____ 14. premolar projection
_____ 15. excessive vertical angulation

Column B

a. patient movement
b. overexposure
c. dimensional distortion
d. elongation
e. long cone technique
f. distal of the canine
g. beam-film alignment
h. film of edentulous area
i. foreshortening
j. inadequate milliamperage
k. film reversal
l. unexposed film area
m. vertical angulation
n. patient tolerance
o. horizontal angulation
p. interproximal caries detection
q. identification dot

IV. Illustrations

1. (Figure 10-1) What error is illustrated here? How would you correct it?

_____
_____
_____

2. (Figure 10-2) What error is illustrated here? How would you correct it?

_____
_____
_____

3. (Figure 10-3) What error is illustrated here? How would you correct it?

_____

_____

_____

4. (Figure 10-4) What error is illustrated here? What would you do to prevent its repetition?

_____

_____

_____

5. (Figure 10-5) What error is illustrated here? What would you do to prevent its repetition?

_____

_____

_____

6. (Figure 10-6) List four possible technique errors that would result in the image shown here.

_____

_____

_____

7. (Figure 10-7) What chairside errors could result in the following film?

_____

_____

_____

V. Complete These Statements

1. In using the paralleling method, the most appropriate FFD is

   _____.

2. An example of a film holder for intraoral periapical radiography is a

   _____ or

   _____.

3. _____ is determined by the area being radiographed, film speed, kilovoltage peak, milliamperage, and FFD.

4. Bitewing radiographs do not show the

   _____.

5. A black, crescent-shaped mark on a radiograph is an indication of

   _____.

6. The occlusal plane of the jaw being radiographed should be

   _____ to the floor.

7. The location on the patient's face that corresponds to the center of the film is called the _____.

8. Failure to align the x-ray beam with the film packet will result in

   _____.

9. If the film packet is curved to accommodate the shape of the palate, it should be curved

   _____ the source of radiation.

10. Another name for the paralleling method is _____.

11. The sagittal plane of the patient's face always should be

    _____.

12. The film packet should be placed

    _____ to both the vertical and horizontal axis of the tooth being radiographed.

13. When taking a full-mouth series, partial dentures always should be

    _____

    _____ to avoid superimposition.

14. Increasing the FFD without changing the milliamperage will result in a

    _____.

15. The most common error in the paralleling technique is in

    _____.

VI. Multiple Choice

Select the best answer.

1. A reason for using the paralleling method instead of the bisecting method is
   a. less thyroid dose to the patient
   b. less dimensional distortion
   c. less exit dose
   d. no superimposition of the zygomatic arch
   e. all of the above

2. Bitewing radiographs are used to detect
   a. periodontal bone loss
   b. interproximal caries
   c. recurrent caries
   d. the ill-fit of metallic restorations
   e. all of the above

3. In taking the radiograph you did not center the beam on the film packet in the patient's mouth. The resulting film will show
   a. fogging
   b. overlapping
   c. elongation
   d. collimator cutoff
   e. foreshortening

4. A set of radiographs all show thin images. One possible error that could have caused this is
   a. the developing solution is too hot
   b. excessive milliampere seconds
   c. excessive kilovoltage peak
   d. excessive FFD
   e. excessive developing time

5. If a film packet is placed in the patient's mouth with the wrong side facing the x-ray beam, the resulting film will
   a. be blank
   b. have a thin image
   c. be overexposed
   d. show no effect
   e. have a thin image with a geometric pattern on it

6. The failure to remove partial dentures while taking radiographs may cause
   a. collimator cutoff
   b. a blurred image
   c. superimposition of the metallic object on the film
   d. overlapped images
   e. double exposure

7. A "long cone" (16-inch FFD) is used in the paralleling technique to
   a. reduce secondary radiation
   b. avoid magnification of the image
   c. avoid distortion of the image
   d. avoid superimposition of the zygomatic arch
   e. facilitate correct vertical angulation

8. Using a localizing ring with a film holder helps in preventing
   a. collimator cutoff
   b. elongation
   c. foreshortening
   d. overlapping
   e. overexposure

9. The projection most likely to excite the gag reflex is the
   a. mandibular molar projection
   b. maxillary molar projection
   c. molar bitewing projection
   d. premolar bitewing projection
   e. maxillary canine projection

10. The best way to prevent patient movement during intraoral radiography is
    a. fast film
    b. short PIDs
    c. good operator technique
    d. high kilovoltage peak
    e. high milliamperage

11. In using a film-holding device with a localizing ring, it is not necessary that
    a. the occlusal plane be parallel to the floor
    b. the sagittal plane be perpendicular to the floor
    c. the backrest be elevated
    d. the headrest be under the occiput
    e. all of the above

12. A full-mouth survey
    a. always has periapical and bitewing films
    b. has a minimum of 20 films
    c. varies in need and number of films according to selection criteria and mouth size
    d. can be replaced in all cases by a panoramic film
    e. none of the above

13. Another correct way to refer to the paralleling method is
    a. short cone technique
    b. right-angle technique
    c. periapical method
    d. bitewing method
    e. none of the above

14. In order to avoid creating an artifact on the apex of the tooth when placing the film in the film holder, which of the following statements is accurate?
    a. "The dot" should be away from "the slot."
    b. "The dot" should be on the opposite the side of "the slot."
    c. It doesn't matter where "the dot" is placed.
    d. "The dot" should be in "the slot."
    e. Placement of "the dot" depends on the projection being taken.

15. Placement of the premolar projection should include
    a. the first and second premolars
    b. most of the first molar
    c. the distal of the canine
    d. only the first and second premolars
    e. a, b, and c

VII. True/False

Select whether each statement is true (**T**) or false (**F**). Circle the correct answer.

1. A bitewing film shows the entire tooth from the occlusal surface or incisal edge to the apex of the tooth. **T/F**
2. The basic principle of the paralleling technique is that the tooth and film should be parallel to each other. **T/F**
3. The use of film holders is strongly discouraged in intraoral radiography. **T/F**
4. The most common exposure error in the paralleling technique is in film placement. **T/F**
5. Blurred images are the result of reversing the film in the patient's mouth. **T/F**

Chapter

11

Accessory Radiographic Techniques: Bisecting Technique and Occlusal Projections

Educational Objectives

After reading Chapter 11 of the textbook and completing this exercise, the student will
1. Understand the geometry of film placement and beam alignment of the bisecting technique.
2. Be able to apply this understanding in the clinical setting and take a full-mouth survey on dentulous and edentulous patients using the bisecting technique.
3. Understand the indications for occlusal radiographs and be able to take these films.

I. Definitions

Define/explain the following terms.

1. Bisecting the angle technique _____

_____

2. Buccolingual dimension _____

_____

3. Dimensional distortion _____

_____

4. Elongated image _____

_____

5. Film plane _____

_____

6. Foreshortened image _____

_____

7. Imaginary bisecting line _____

_____

8. Headrest position _____

_____

9. Horizontal angulation _____

_____

10. Negative angulation _____

_____

11. Occlusal film packet _____

_____

12. Occlusal plane orientation _____

_____

13. Occlusal projection _____

_____

14. Overlapped image _____

_____

15. Positive angulation _____

_____

16. Right-angle occlusal projection _____

_____

17. Sagittal plane orientation _____

_____

18. Short cone _____

_____

19. Topographic occlusal projection _____

_____

20. Vertical angulation _____

_____

II. Comprehension Exercise

1. Describe the advantages of the bisecting technique as compared to the paralleling technique.

2. What generally is the indication for use of an occlusal projection? What are the specific indications for topographic versus right-angle projections?

3. Describe the disadvantages of the bisecting technique when compared to the paralleling technique.

4. Describe the method used with the bisecting-angle technique.

5. Explain the difference between horizontal angulation and vertical angulation. What does each determine?

6. In the bisecting technique, what dictates the point of entry?

7. Why is the thyroid dose higher in the bisecting technique than in the paralleling technique?

8. In intraoral radiography, what is the correct sagittal plane orientation for the patient's head?

9. Why does the bisecting technique call for an 8-inch focal-film distance (FFD)?

10. In the bisecting technique, what determines the variations in vertical angulation from one projection to another?

11. Explain why it is necessary to use occlusal projections when localizing impacted teeth.

12. In an edentulous survey, what is the main reason for using topographic occlusal films? Name two alternatives.

13. Why is the use of shorter exposure times with the bisecting technique not valid as an advantage at this point in time?

14. In the bisecting technique, why is occlusal plane orientation so critical?

15. Explain why the topographic occlusal projection is said to be a modification of the bisecting technique.

III. Matching

Match the items in *Column A* with the appropriate items in *Column B*.

Column A

_____ 1. elongation
_____ 2. buccolingual localization
_____ 3. 8-inch FFD
_____ 4. poor sagittal plane orientation
_____ 5. foreshortening
_____ 6. higher thyroid dose
_____ 7. occlusal plane
_____ 8. overlapped image
_____ 9. greater exit dose
_____ 10. short buccal image structure
_____ 11. dimensional accuracy
_____ 12. large pathologic areas
_____ 13. positive angulation
_____ 14. negative angulation
_____ 15. #4 size film

Column B

a. bisecting technique
b. parallel to the floor
c. dimensional distortion
d. topographic occlusal
e. poor horizontal angulation
f. image magnification
g. insufficient vertical angulation
h. occlusal film size
i. too much vertical angulation
j. periapical film size
k. right-angle occlusal projection
l. mandibular arch
m. fogged image
n. elongation
o. maxillary arch
p. 8-inch FFD
q. paralleling technique

IV. Illustrations

1. Draw the correct relationship of the central ray, teeth, and film in a diagram of horizontal angulation using the bisecting technique as compared with the paralleling technique.

2. Diagram the relationship of the central ray, tooth, and film packet for the bisecting technique.

3. (Figure 11-1) Which of these maxillary molar periapical films, A or B, was taken with the paralleling technique? Which was taken with the bisecting technique?

A

B

a. _____

b. _____

4. (Figure 11-2) What error was made here? What caused it?

5. (Figure 11-3) Was too little or too much vertical angulation used to produce this radiograph? What error is the result?

_____

_____

_____

_____

_____

_____

6. (Figure 11-4) Identify the error seen here, and explain how you would correct it.

_____

_____

_____

7. (Figure 11-5) In this film taken with the bisecting technique, how would you describe the image? What technique error caused it?

_____

_____

_____

V. Complete These Statements

1. The projection of choice to completely visualize a palatal lesion would be _____.

2. The dose to the thyroid gland is _____ in the bisecting technique when compared to the paralleling technique because of _____.

3. The correct chair position for the bisecting technique requires that the sagittal plane of the patient's face is _____ to the floor.

4. The anatomic landmark for the point of entry for the mandibular bicuspid periapical film is the _____.

5. Periodontal bone height may be exaggerated in the bisecting technique because of _____.

6. In the bisecting technique an overly dense film may be caused by _____ or _____.

7. Foreshortening can be caused by excessive vertical angulation or poor _____ orientation.

8. Two projections other than periapical films that can be used in an edentulous survey of the mandible are _____ and _____.

9. Usually the FFD used in the paralleling technique is _____ than in the bisecting technique.

10. The major disadvantage of the bisecting technique is that the image projected on the film is _____.

11. The vertical angulation for the maxillary incisors in the bisecting technique would be about _____ degrees.

12. In the bisecting technique the film packet should be held in the patient's mouth with a _____.

13. Horizontal angulation is established so that the _____ is perpendicular to the film in the _____ plane.

14. Occlusal film has the _____ speed (sensitivity) as periapical film size #2.

15. The angulation of the _____ may vary from 45 to 75 degrees, depending on the anatomic area.

VI. Multiple Choice

Select the best answer.

1. You have decided to change the PID in your office, replacing the 16-inch cylinder with an 8-inch cylinder. The milliamperage will remain the same, as will the kilovolt peak value. The old exposure time for mandibular molars was 36 impulses; the new exposure time to obtain films of equal density will be
   a. 12 impulses
   b. 24 impulses
   c. 18 impulses
   d. 9 impulses
   e. 48 impulses

2. The posterior topographic view of the maxilla can be considered a topographic view of the
   a. zygoma
   b. maxillary sinus
   c. zygomatic process
   d. maxillary tuberosity
   e. none of the above

3. In taking a periapical radiograph using the bisecting technique, the x-ray beam was not centered on the film packet. The resulting film shows
   a. fogging
   b. overlapping
   c. collimator cutoff
   d. foreshortening
   e. elongation

4. In taking a periapical radiograph of the maxillary incisor area by the bisecting technique, using a vertical angulation of +15 degrees will result in a film that
   a. has collimator cutoff
   b. is foreshortened
   c. is elongated
   d. is overlapped
   e. is correct

5. When using the bisecting-angle technique for a maxillary premolar projection, the point of entry is
   a. the base of the lateral nasal groove
   b. just below the midpoint of the nares
   c. the most anterior part of the cheekbone
   d. the zygomatic arch
   e. none of the above

6. The best way to visualize a salivary stone in the floor of the mouth is by using
   a. panoramic projection
   b. maxillary occlusal projection
   c. mandibular central incisor projection
   d. mandibular right-angle occlusal projection
   e. mandibular topographic occlusal projection

7. Occlusal film is classified as size
   a. #2
   b. #0
   c. #4
   d. #3
   e. #1

8. For the maxillary molar periapical projection, the center of the film packet should be aligned with
   a. the junction between the first and second molars
   b. the middle of the first molar
   c. the junction between the second and third molars
   d. the middle of the second molar
   e. none of the above

9. In the bisecting technique, if the central ray is not perpendicular to the film packet in the horizontal plane, the resulting film will be
   a. foreshortened
   b. overlapped
   c. "cone cut"
   d. elongated
   e. blurred

10. Using the bisecting technique in taking a periapical radiograph of tooth #32, using a vertical angulation of −30 degrees will result in a film that is
    a. foreshortened
    b. overlapped
    c. elongated
    d. "cone cut"
    e. reversed

11. What would be the projection of choice to visualize a large lesion in the midline of the palate?
    a. panoramic
    b. maxillary right-angle occlusal
    c. maxillary topographic occlusal
    d. maxillary molar periapical
    e. maxillary incisor periapical

12. When using the bisecting technique, the point of entry for the mandibular molar projection is the
   a. roots of the molars
   b. root of the first molar
   c. cemento-enamel junction of the molars
   d. crowns of the molars
   e. bifurcation of the second molar

13. The film speed of occlusal film is
   a. slower than periapical film
   b. the same as periapical film
   c. faster than bitewing film
   d. the same as panoramic film
   e. faster than periapical film

14. The best projection to decide whether an impacted maxillary cuspid is located bucally or lingually is the
   a. maxillary topographic occlusal
   b. panoramic
   c. cuspid periapical using the paralleling method
   d. cuspid periapical using the bisecting method
   e. maxillary right-angle occlusal

15. The bisecting-angle technique may be an advantageous technique to use with
   a. small children
   b. people with low palatal vaults
   c. patients with small mouths
   d. patients with anatomic constraints prohibiting the use of paralleling devices
   e. all of the above

VII. True/False

Select whether each statement is true (**T**) or false (**F**). Circle the correct answer.

1. In the bisecting technique, the film is placed parallel to the occlusal surfaces of the teeth being radiographed. **T/F**
2. The major disadvantage of the bisecting technique is dimensional inaccuracy. **T/F**
3. In the bisecting technique, the central ray is directed perpendicular to an imaginary bisecting line between the tooth and film. **T/F**
4. Foreshortening is a result of overbending of the film packet in the bisecting technique. **T/F**
5. Occlusal radiographs are seldom taken to view salivary stones in the submandibular gland. **T/F**

Chapter
12

Panoramic Radiography

I. Definitions

Define/explain the following terms.

1. Ala-tragus line _____

_____

2. Digital imaging _____

_____

3. Electrostatic artifact _____

_____

4. Focal trough _____

_____

5. Frankfort horizontal plane _____

_____

6. Ghost image _____

_____

7. Image layer _____

_____

8. Midsagittal plane _____

_____

9. Panoramic radiography _____

_____

10. "Panorex" _____

_____

11. Pantomograph _____

_____

12. Point of rotation _____

_____

13. Slit beam _____

_____

14. Tomographic cut _____

_____

15. Tomography _____

_____

II. Comprehension Exercise

1. What are the advantages of a panoramic radiograph when compared to a full-mouth intraoral survey?

2. What are the disadvantages of a panoramic radiograph when compared to a full-mouth intraoral survey?

3. What does the term panorama mean? What is the term's significance in panoramic radiography?

4. Why is patient jaw position so important in panoramic radiography?

5. How is patient movement avoided in panoramic radiography?

6. What are the two techniques available that produce panoramic films? Which technique is more widely used? Why?

7. What special precautions are necessary when processing panoramic films?

8. In panoramic radiography, what is a ghost image? How can it be avoided?

9. How can panoramic units be used to take tomograms of the temporomandibular joint (TMJ)?

10. What is the focal trough?

11. What is a "computer-driven tomographic unit"?

12. What is the main indication for panoramic radiographs?

13. What is a tomographic "slice" or "cut?"

14. Why are panoramic radiographs not recommended for caries detection and periodontal bone evaluation?

15. Is digital imaging available for panoramic units? If so, explain the basic principles involved.

III. Matching

Match the items in *Column A* with the appropriate items in *Column B*.

Column A

_____ 1. rare earth elements
_____ 2. tomogram
_____ 3. focal trough
_____ 4. static marks
_____ 5. circular tube motion
_____ 6. thyroid collar
_____ 7. tongue position
_____ 8. patient movement
_____ 9. mandibular condyle
_____ 10. intraoral x-ray source
_____ 11. open and closed view
_____ 12. slouching patient
_____ 13. tomographic series
_____ 14. first panoramic unit
_____ 15. ghost image

Column B

a. plane of acceptable detail
b. TMJ tomography
c. Panorex
d. tightly packed film
e. objects with high density
f. radiopaque triangle
g. seen on pantomograms
h. not used for pantomograms
i. thyroid collar
j. multiple cuts
k. pharyngeal air space
l. rotating anode
m. blurred image
n. intensifying screen
o. laminogram
p. tomogram
q. distorted image

IV. Illustrations

1. (Figure 12-1) What error is shown here?

_____

_____

2. (Figure 12-2) What error was made here?

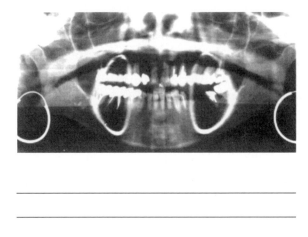

_____

_____

_____

3. (Figure 12-3) What error was made here?

_____

_____

_____

4. (Figure 12-4) What error was made here?

_____

_____

_____

5. (Figure 12-5) What error was made here?

_____

_____

_____

6. (Figure 12-6) What is the circular radiopaque structure in the right posterior maxilla?

_____

_____

_____

V. Complete These Statements

1. Three anatomic landmarks seen on panoramic films that do not appear on intraoral full-mouth series are the

   _____,

   _____, and

   _____.

2. The area of the maxilla that is seen with least amount of definition on a panoramic radiograph is the

   _____.

3. The panoramic image does not have the same _____ that is seen on intraoral periapical or bitewing film.

4. The main advantage of a panoramic radiograph over intraoral periapical films is the _____.

5. The bilateral radiolucent structures seen crossing the ramus of the mandible on panoramic radiographs are the _____.

6. Multiple black linear streaks on a panoramic radiograph are a result of _____.

7. Another name for the "plane of acceptable detail" is the _____.

8. In comparing patient radiation dose, panoramic radiographs require _____ radiation than a full-mouth series.

9. In panoramic radiography, the midsagittal plane should be _____ to the floor and the _____ plane and the _____ line should be _____ to the floor for correct patient positioning.

10. When taking a panoramic radiograph the patient's tongue should always be _____.

_____

11. The main disadvantage of panoramic films when compared to a full-mouth survey is _____.

12. A lead apron should be used without a _____ for panoramic radiography.

13. A recently reported use of panoramic films is the detection of _____

_____ in the patient's neck region.

14. An image from the other side of the patient's jaw that is seen as a blurred shadow is called a _____ image.

15. The most skilled operator requires at least 15 to 20 minutes to perform an intraoral survey; pantomographs can be taken in less than _____.

VI. Multiple Choice

Select the best answer.

1. When taking a pantomogram, the patient's lead apron should
   a. be placed in the usual manner
   b. not be used at all
   c. be placed on the back of the patient
   d. not be placed lower than the clavicles
   e. be placed over the thyroid area

2. Object scatter degrading the image is not a concern in panoramic radiography
   a. because of the rotation of the tube head
   b. because of the narrow slit beam
   c. because of the inherent filtration
   d. because the patient is seated
   e. because of the intensifying screens

3. In positioning a patient for panoramic radiography, if the patient's head is tilted up
   a. a right oblique (RO) triangle is seen in the mandibular anterior region
   b. a radiolucent (RL) line is seen above the apices of the maxillary teeth
   c. the chin is back and the forehead is forward
   d. the RO palate is superimposed over the apices of the upper teeth
   e. the lower anterior teeth appear narrow and blurred

4. Each successive panoramic film appears lighter than the one before. Which of the following corrections should be made?
   a. increase the mA setting
   b. increase the kVp setting
   c. change the intensifying screen
   d. change the developer solution
   e. reduce the temperature of the developer

5. Which of the following anatomic structures is usually not seen on intraoral periapical radiographs but is seen on pantomograms?
   a. mental foramen
   b. mandibular foramen
   c. mylohyoid ridge
   d. coronoid process
   e. median palatal suture

6. If the lead apron is placed too high on the patient,
   a. it will create a large RL on the film
   b. it will create a large RO on the film
   c. it will create an RO on the maxilla
   d. it will obliterate all the mandibular teeth
   e. it will create a vertical RL line on the film

7. The main reason for taking a panoramic radiograph would be
   a. to lower the patient's exposure
   b. to see the borders of a lesion that are larger than periapical film
   c. that it requires less time
   d. for better object definition
   e. the film cost

8. Grids are usually not used with panoramic units because
   a. there is no object scatter
   b. the moving field size is very narrow
   c. the motion makes grids ineffective
   d. the film is too sensitive
   e. the mA setting is not high enough

9. Panoramic radiographs cannot be used for detection of
   a. impacted teeth
   b. jaw fractures
   c. caries and periodontal disease
   d. large areas of pathology
   e. eruption patterns

10. In taking a tomographic series, the depth of "cuts" can be varied by
    a. varying the focal object distance
    b. changing the kVp setting
    c. varying the mA setting
    d. changing the type of motion
    e. increasing the exposure time

11. The main advantage of using an intraoral source for panoramic radiography is
    a. better tooth definition
    b. less image distortion
    c. no film is necessary
    d. significant reduction in patient radiation dose
    e. less image magnification

12. Common positioning requirements for panoramic units include
    a. the anterior teeth are positioned in the proper groove in the bite block
    b. the ala-tragus line should be parallel to the floor
    c. the midsagittal plane should be perpendicular to the floor
    d. the chin should not be angled up or down
    e. all of the above

13. In positioning the patient for a pantomographic radiograph, if the patient is too far forward
    a. the hard palate will be superimposed on the maxillary anteriors
    b. the upper and lower anterior teeth will be blurred
    c. the film cassette will hit the patient's head
    d. the posterior teeth will be blurred
    e. there will be a radiolucent streak on the film

14. The use of rare earth intensifying screens in pantomographic units
    a. is not possible
    b. is not necessary
    c. is recommended
    d. would not decrease the radiation dose to the brain
    e. would not decrease the radiation dose to the thyroid

15. Advantages of panoramic radiography include all of the following *except*
    a. less time
    b. better patient cooperation
    c. overuse
    d. lower bone marrow dose
    e. simple to perform

VII. True/False

Select whether each statement is true (**T**) or false (**F**). Circle the correct answer.

1. A panoramic radiograph is produced by moving the film and x-ray source in the same direction around the patient. **T/F**

2. Most of the errors in panoramic radiography are as a result of poor patient positioning. **T/F**

3. If the patient is positioned too far forward, the lower anterior teeth will appear blurred and widened. **T/F**

4. The main indication for panoramic radiography is attaining a larger field size than is possible with periapical radiography. **T/F**

5. Ghosting will occur if static electricity is caused during processing of panoramic film. **T/F**

Chapter

13

Extraoral Techniques

Educational Objectives

After reading Chapter 13 of the textbook and completing this exercise, the student will
1. Understand the indications for extraoral projections and be able to apply them in clinical practice.
2. Understand the use of intensifying screens and grids and their clinical importance.
3. Be able to take the extraoral projections discussed in the chapter.

I. Definitions

Define/explain the following terms.

1. Cassette _____

_____

2. Cephalometric radiography _____

_____

3. Extraoral projection _____

_____

4. Film-holding board _____

_____

5. Grid _____

_____

6. Lateral oblique projection _____

_____

7. Lateral skull projection _____

_____

8. Object scatter _____

_____

9. Submentovertex (SMV) projection _____

_____

10. Waters projection _____

_____

II. Comprehension Exercise

1. Describe three clinical indications for using extraoral films in dentistry.

2. Which extraoral projection is most diagnostic for pathologic conditions of the maxillary sinus? How is this film taken?

3. What type of x-ray unit is used for taking extraoral radiographs?

4. What special precautions must be taken in the darkroom when loading cassettes and processing extraoral films?

5. What are the advantages of using rare earth intensifying screens?

6. What equipment is needed for taking standard extraoral projections?

7. How can you identify the right and left sides in addition to labeling patient information on extraoral film?

8. Explain how and why the film-screen system is used in extraoral radiography.

9. How can one differentiate the left side of the patient from the right on an extraoral radiograph?

10. How does the use of intensifying screens reduce the exposure needed for radiographs?

11. What six factors should be known for every extraoral projection?

12. If a periapical film of an impacted mandibular third molar cannot be positioned so that the complete root can be seen, what would you do?

13. What is object scatter?

14. What is the lateral oblique projection of the mandible used to survey? Why is this projection ideal for visualizing?

15. Why are grids not necessary in periapical, bitewing, and panoramic radiographs?

16. Why do you need a minimum of 36 inches focal-film distance (FFD) for a lateral skull projection?

17. What are the advantages of an extraoral film holder over the patient holding the cassette?

18. Why are grids used in extraoral projections and not for intraoral film?

19. What does varying mA and kVp settings depend on in extraoral radiography?

III. Matching

Match the items in *Column A* with the appropriate items in *Column B*.

Column A

_____ 1. grid
_____ 2. lateral skull projection
_____ 3. rigid cassette
_____ 4. thyroid collar
_____ 5. midline fracture of mandible
_____ 6. left and right side
_____ 7. minimum safelight
_____ 8. posteroanterior projection
_____ 9. lateral oblique projection
_____ 10. Waters projection
_____ 11. reduce patient exposure
_____ 12. cephalostat
_____ 13. submentovertex
_____ 14. point of entry
_____ 15. fogged film

Column B

a. fractures of the cheekbone
b. improper safelight
c. processing extraoral film
d. articular disc
e. external auditory meatus
f. extraoral projection
g. head positioning
h. cephalometric
i. posteroanterior projection
j. need lead marker
k. maxillary sinusitis
l. position with forehead and nose against cassette
m. intensifying screens
n. object scatter
o. fractured mandible
p. film packet
q. not used in extraoral radiography

IV. Illustrations

1. (Figure 13-1) Identify this radiographic projection.

_____

_____

_____

2. Draw a schematic of the radiographic technique used for the projection in Figure 13-1.

3. (Figure 13-2) Identify this radiographic projection.

_____

_____

_____

4. Draw a schematic of the radiographic technique used for the projection in Figure 13-2.

5. (Figure 13-3) Identify this radiographic projection.

_____

_____

_____

6. Draw a schematic of the radiographic technique used for the projection in Figure 13-3.

7. Make a drawing that illustrates the use of a grid in dental radiography.

8. (Figure 13-4) Identify this radiographic projection.

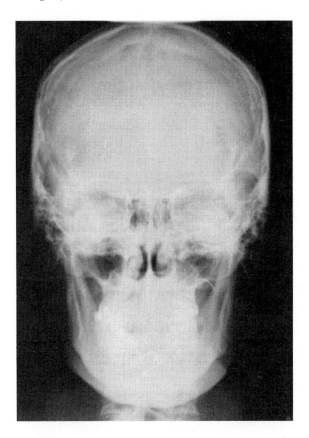

_____

_____

_____

9. (Figure 13-5) What radiographic projection is seen here? Be specific!

_____

_____

_____

10. (Figure 13-6) What radiographic projection is seen here? Be specific!

_____

_____

_____

V. Complete These Statements

1. When comparing radiographic detail, it can be said that film-screen combinations produce _____ detail when compared with film alone.

2. Some states have statutes that _____ or _____ certain members of the dental health team from performing specific extraoral radiographic techniques.

3. Patients who have _____ or _____ _____ cannot open their mouths and would benefit from an extraoral radiographic series.

4. The extraoral projection that is most diagnostic for the maxillary sinus is the _____.

5. The two extraoral projections that are needed to visualize a fracture of the angle of the mandible are _____ and _____.

6. Orthodontists would most likely use the _____ for cephalometric measurements.

7. In extraoral radiography the field size is _____ than in intraoral radiography.

8. The lateral skull projection would not be used to visualize a large mandibular cyst because of _____ _____.

9. The _____ provides a means of localizing changes in a mediolateral direction.

10. Grids are not used in panoramic radiography because _____ _____.

11. Extraoral films are processed _____ as intraoral films.

12. The increased FFD utilized in extraoral radiography is necessary to get a sufficiently large _____ at the patient's face.

13. In both the lateral skull and posterior anterior projections, the sagittal plane of the patient's skull is _____ to the floor.

14. For the lateral skull projection, the central ray is directed at the _____.

15. The _____ projection is used to visualize the sphenoid and ethmoid sinuses.

VI. Multiple Choice

Select the best answer.

1. The best extraoral projection for viewing an impacted left mandibular third molar is
   a. submental vertex
   b. posterior anterior
   c. left lateral oblique
   d. lateral skull
   e. right lateral oblique

2. Grids are used to
   a. mark films
   b. reduce background radiation
   c. reduce field size
   d. collimate the x-ray beam
   e. reduce object scatter

3. In extraoral radiography, an increased FFD is necessary to
   a. decrease patient exposure
   b. increase the beam divergence
   c. decrease the beam divergence
   d. increase film quality
   e. decrease image magnification

4. The best way to visualize maxillary sinus pathology using a dental x-ray machine is a
   a. lateral oblique projection
   b. maxillary occlusal projection
   c. posterior anterior projection
   d. transcranial projection
   e. Waters projection

5. In taking a Waters projection the patient's
   a. head is inclined 15 degrees
   b. nose and chin touch the cassette, mouth open
   c. nose and chin touch the cassette, mouth closed
   d. forehead and nose touch the cassette, mouth open
   e. forehead and chin touch the cassette

6. Extraoral cassettes
   a. may be rigid or flexible
   b. contain intensifying screens
   c. are light-tight
   d. are available in varying sizes
   e. all of the above

7. If all of your extraoral films appear dense and fogged after processing while your intraoral films are satisfactory, the probable cause is
   a. the solutions are too hot
   b. white light exposure in the darkroom
   c. the safelight is too intense
   d. the safelight is too weak
   e. the solutions are exhausted

8. Extraoral films are processed
   a. only with automatic processors
   b. by the time-temperature method
   c. by sight development
   d. with special solutions
   e. none of the above

9. Holding devices have the advantage
   a. of preventing a fogged film
   b. of standardizing techniques
   c. preventing patient and film movement
   d. Both a and c are acceptable answers.
   e. Both b and c are acceptable answers.

10. A fractured zygomatic arch can be seen on a(an)
    a. lateral oblique projection
    b. posteroanterior projection
    c. Waters projection
    d. anteroposterior projection
    e. lateral skull projection

11. The major disadvantage of using extraoral projections with screens in dentistry is
    a. the cost of the equipment
    b. problems with processing
    c. an increased radiation dose
    d. decreased definition
    e. operative difficulty

12. The screen film used in extraoral radiography is
    a. more sensitive to light
    b. more sensitive to radiation
    c. equally sensitive to both light and radiation
    d. not changed by light or radiation
    e. none of the above are significant statements

13. A pathologic condition in the midline of the mandible can best be diagnosed using
    a. a right lateral oblique projection
    b. a lateral skull projection
    c. a left lateral oblique projection
    d. a Waters projection
    e. a posteroanterior projection

14. The lateral oblique projection of the mandible is not diagnostic anterior to the canine because of the superimposition caused by
    a. the mental ridges
    b. the mental eminence
    c. the genial tubercles
    d. the anterior curve of the mandible
    e. the lingual foramen

15. Exposure, mA, and kVp settings vary with extraoral radiographs depending on the
    a. film speed
    b. intensifying screen
    c. size of the patient
    d. None of the above are possible answers.
    e. All of the above are possible answers.

VII. True/False

Select whether each statement is true (**T**) or false (**F**). Circle the correct answer.

1. Some states have statutes that prohibit or limit the dental professional from performing certain extraoral techniques. **T/F**
2. Extraoral screen films are less sensitive to light than are intraoral films. **T/F**
3. The lateral oblique projection of the mandible is used for viewing mandibular third molar impactions and pathology. **T/F**
4. Waters view of the maxillary sinuses is used for maxillary sinus pathologic conditions and facial fractures of the upper third of the face. **T/F**
5. For the submentovertex projection, the central ray is directed from beneath the chin at 45° to the cassette. **T/F**

Chapter

14

Radiography of the Temporomandibular Joint

Educational Objectives

After reading Chapter 14 of the textbook and completing this exercise, the student will
1. Know and understand the imaging techniques available for viewing the temporomandibular joint (TMJ).

I. Definitions

Define/explain the following terms.

1. Arthritic changes _____

   _____

2. Articular disc _____

   _____

3. Arthrography _____

   _____

4. Basaler projection _____

   _____

5. Computed tomography (CT) _____

   _____

6. Contrast medium _____

   _____

7. External auditory meatus _____

   _____

8. Magnetic resonance imaging (MRI) _____

   _____

9. Positioning board _____

   _____

10. Transcranial technique _____

    _____

II. Comprehension Exercise

1. Discuss the use of conventional tomography in TMJ radiography.

2. How is a contrast medium used in articular disc imaging?

3. Which anatomic structures of the TMJ cannot be seen with routine radiographic imaging?

4. List the pathologic conditions of the TMJ that may be visible on radiographs.

5. Why should dental professionals feel comfortable in dealing with radiographic images of the TMJ?

6. Explain the advantage of using CT in TMJ radiography.

7. Briefly describe the transcranial imaging technique used in viewing the TMJ.

8. What is the advantage of using positioning boards in the transcranial imaging technique?

9. Which anatomic structures of the TMJ should be identifiable on radiographs?

10. Why is MRI very effective in viewing the articular disc of the TMJ? Explain.

III. Matching

Match the items in *Column A* with the appropriate items in *Column B*.

Column A

_____ 1. CT
_____ 2. articular disc
_____ 3. TMJ pathology
_____ 4. MRI
_____ 5. panoramic radiograph
_____ 6. positioning device
_____ 7. weak signal
_____ 8. strong signal
_____ 9. submentovertex (SMV) projection
_____ 10. arthrography

Column B

a. soft tissue imaging
b. entire maxilla and mandible
c. axial plane
d. meniscus
e. lateral skull projection
f. high density
g. opaque contrast medium
h. ankylosis
i. cephalometric radiograph
j. low density
k. viewing in three planes
l. transcranial technique

IV. Illustrations

1. Draw a diagram of the normal temporomandibular joint and label all essential components.

2. (Figure 14-1) Identify all the essential components in the tomogram of the TMJ.

V. Complete These Statements

1. Patients with symptoms relating to the _____ are not uncommon in dental practice.

2. _____ is very effective for viewing the articular disc.

3. In _____ the articular disc is outlined with an opaque contrast medium.

4. CT enables viewing of an area in _____ planes.

5. The _____ projection can also be used as a scout film for tomograms of the TMJ.

6. The internal and external _____ muscles are not seen on radiographs.

7. Since the TMJ is a movable structure, the condyle should be viewed in _____ positions.

8. The joint is anatomically bound laterally by the _____ arch.

9. Before the wide use of CT in TMJ imaging, _____ was used to examine the condyles radiographically.

10. The TMJ is anatomically bound medially by the _____ of the temporal bone.

VI. Multiple Choice

Select the best answer.

1. Which of the following imaging techniques is considered invasive and may result in related complications?
   a. CT
   b. MRI
   c. SMV projection
   d. arthrography
   e. none of the above

2. Pathology of the TMJ that can be visible on radiographs may include
   a. disc displacement
   b. fibrous adhesions
   c. malignant tumors
   d. a and b only
   e. all of the above

3. The most important reason for using an angling board in transcranial radiography of the TMJ is
   a. it is easier
   b. less radiation is used
   c. open and closed positions can be compared accurately
   d. it saves film
   e. none of the above

4. Of the following, which method is most effective in producing diagnostic images of the articular disc?
   a. MRI
   b. conventional tomography
   c. CT
   d. panoramic radiography
   e. none of the above

5. The cassette used when producing four views of the TMJ is usually a
   a. 5 × 7 inch cassette
   b. 5 × 12 inch cassette
   c. 8 × 13 inch cassette
   d. 8 × 10 inch cassette
   e. none of the above

6. A conventional panoramic radiograph will show both the right and left joints in
   a. the sagittal plane
   b. the frontal plane
   c. the occlusal plane
   d. the lateral plane
   e. all of the above

7. On a magnetic resonance image of the TMJ, the articular disc will appear
   a. opaque
   b. lucent
   c. mixed
   d. radiopaque
   e. none of the above

8. On a radiograph, the fibrocartilage associated with the TMJ will appear
   a. RO
   b. RL
   c. opaque
   d. mixed
   e. none of the above

9. Which structures of the TMJ will appear radiopaque on a radiograph?
   a. the condyles, articular disc, and meniscus
   b. the glenoid fossa, cartilage, and articular fossa
   c. the condyles, neck of the condyles, and articular eminence
   d. the internal and external pterygoid muscles
   e. none of the above

10. In which three positions should the TMJ be viewed?
    a. open, shifted right, and shifted left
    b. closed, shifted right, and shifted left
    c. open, closed, rest
    d. closed, rest, slightly open
    e. none of the above

VII. True/False

Select whether each statement is true (**T**) or false (**F**). Circle the correct answer.

1. Patients with TMJ symptoms are very uncommon in dental practice. **T/F**
2. The articular disc is a minor source of TMJ disorders. **T/F**
3. Some panoramic units have specific programs for the TMJ that will also allow one to take views in the open and closed positions. **T/F**
4. Before the wide use of CT scanning, conventional tomography was one of the better ways to examine the condyle radiographically. **T/F**
5. Arthrography is an invasive procedure that may have complications. **T/F**

Chapter

15 Digital Imaging

Educational Objectives

After reading Chapter 15 of the textbook and completing this exercise, the student will

1. Understand the principles of digital imaging and how they can be used in the dental office.
2. Be able to produce images using digital radiography.

I. Definitions

Define/explain the following terms.

1. Analogue signal _____

_____

2. Charged coupling device (CCD) _____

_____

3. Complementary metal oxide semiconductor (CMOS) _____

_____

4. Detector _____

_____

5. Digital image _____

_____

6. Digitize _____

_____

7. Direct digital radiography _____

_____

8. Electronic sensor _____

_____

9. Gray level _____

_____

10. Hard copy _____

_____

11. Image manipulation _____
_____

12. Imaging plate _____
_____

13. Optical scanning _____
_____

14. Pixel _____
_____

15. Storage _____
_____

16. Phosphor _____
_____

II. Comprehension Exercise

1. What are the advantages of intraoral digital imaging in comparison with film?

2. What are the disadvantages of intraoral digital imaging in comparison with film?

3. What is the basic concept behind digital radiography? When and by whom was it introduced into dentistry?

4. Explain the difference between direct and indirect digital imaging.

5. Why does digital radiography produce less patient exposure to radiation than film?

6. What are the basic elements necessary to acquire a digital image?

7. Explain the difference between indirect digital radiography and optical scanning.

8. How is image definition measured? How does definition in digital radiography compare to film definition?

9. What are the three basic types of digital imaging systems?

10. What are gray levels?

11. Why is digital radiography described as environmentally friendly?

12. Name the three most common sensors employed in digital radiography. State the basic differences among the three.

13. Can the digital image be manipulated to show a third plane (axial)? If not, why not?

14. What is remote consultation? How does it apply to digital radiography?

15. What advantage of digital radiography is most appealing to dentists? Why?

III. Matching

Match the items in *Column A* with the appropriate items in *Column B*.

Column A

_____ 1. RVG
_____ 2. optical scanning
_____ 3. sensor
_____ 4. storage phosphor
_____ 5. digitize
_____ 6. gray levels
_____ 7. digital image definition
_____ 8. image storage
_____ 9. patient exposure
_____ 10. instant image acquisition
_____ 11. digital radiography
_____ 12. pixels
_____ 13. hard copies
_____ 14. image manipulation

Column B

a. laser scan
b. 256
c. processed radiographs
d. computer
e. group D film
f. "filmless radiography"
g. first dental digital unit
h. admissible in court
i. containers for numbers
j. convert to numbers
k. printouts
l. film processing
m. group E film
n. direct digital image
o. 9 to 10 line pairs per millimeter
p. charged coupling device (CCD)
q. 60% reduction

IV. Complete These Statements

1. Two types of sensors used in direct digital radiography are

   _____ and

   _____ .

2. When compared with D-speed film, digital radiography results in an exposure decrease of _____%.

3. When compared with E-speed film, digital radiography results in an exposure decrease of _____%.

4. In the storage phosphor unit the sensor is scanned by a _____ .

5. A digital image is composed of discrete areas called _____ .

6. Once acquired, the computer can change the _____ in many ways.

7. The human eye can only discern about _____ gray levels.

8. Digital images can be stored in a

   _____ .

9. Images taken at different times can be placed on the monitor side by side for

   _____ .

10. Digital images can be sent to an insurance company by _____ or by making a

    _____ .

11. In both direct and indirect digital radiography a _____ is not needed.

12. Because the silver salts found in film emulsion and processing chemicals are not used in digital imaging, there are no _____ and _____ issues.

13. In direct digital radiography the image appears on the screen _____.

14. In direct digital radiography the sensor is thicker and more _____ than in indirect digital radiography.

15. The main disadvantage of digital imaging is _____.

V. Multiple Choice

Select the best answer.

1. The standard dental x-ray unit
   a. cannot be used for digital radiography
   b. is not capable of producing the short exposure time needed for digital radiography
   c. can be used for digital radiography
   d. is not capable of producing the long exposures needed
   e. none of the above

2. The storage phosphor sensor is
   a. larger than direct sensors
   b. more rigid than direct sensors
   c. more sensitive than direct sensors
   d. thinner than direct sensors
   e. none of the above

3. The type of digital imaging system that is similar to scanning a document is
   a. direct digital radiography
   b. optically scanned digital radiography
   c. indirect digital radiography
   d. direct digital scanning
   e. indirect digital scanning

4. The human eye can discern about
   a. 9 to 10 gray levels
   b. 256 gray levels
   c. 100 gray levels
   d. 32 gray levels
   e. 100 gray levels

5. Darkroom and processing capability is needed in
   a. direct digital radiography
   b. optical scanning digital radiography
   c. storage phosphor technique
   d. indirect digital radiography
   e. none of the above

6. The most critical part of a digital radiographic system is the
   a. computer
   b. printer
   c. scanner
   d. sensor
   e. software

7. Digital imaging for panoramic units
   a. is now available
   b. cannot be done
   c. is not yet available
   d. increases the patient exposure
   e. needs standard processing

8. A "hard copy" is
   a. a duplicate radiograph
   b. an image that is hard to acquire
   c. a computer printout
   d. a rigid radiograph
   e. none of the above

9. The digital image has
   a. 4 to 8 line pairs per millimeter
   b. 9 to 10 line pairs per millimeter
   c. 12 to 15 line pairs per millimeter
   d. 13 to 16 line pairs per millimeter
   e. 17 to 20 line pairs per millimeter

10. When compared to D-speed film, digital radiography can reduce the patient's exposure by
    a. 60%
    b. 90%
    c. 150%
    d. 200%
    e. none of the above

11. In direct digital radiography, a digital image can be generated in anywhere from
    a. 1 to 3 minutes
    b. 1.5 to 3 minutes
    c. 1 to 4 minutes
    d. 1.5 to 4.5 minutes
    e. 1.5 to 5 minutes

12. The major difficulty in using direct digital radiography is
    a. using the bisecting technique
    b. placing the sensor parallel to the tooth
    c. patient movement
    d. time consumed
    e. radiation exposure

13. Digital images
    a. can be integrated into an office record system
    b. can be enlarged
    c. can be inverted
    d. can be colorized
    e. all of the above

14. Digital intraoral sensors are
    a. autoclavable
    b. extremely sturdy
    c. available in only one size
    d. quite fragile
    e. none of the above

15. All of the digital imaging systems differ in how they
    a. acquire the digital image
    b. transmit the image
    c. display the image
    d. adjust the image
    e. store the image

VI. True/False

Select whether each statement is true (**T**) or false (**F**). Circle the correct answer.

1. The most critical part of a digital radiography system is the sensor that is placed in the patient's mouth. **T/F**
2. A digital image is composed of structurally ordered areas called analogues. **T/F**
3. In a direct digital radiography system, the sensor is connected by a wire to the computer. **T/F**
4. Indirect digital radiography employs the use of storage phosphor plates directly connected to the computer. **T/F**
5. In optically scanned digital radiography systems, regular dental film is used to acquire the image. **T/F**

Chapter

16

Advanced Imaging Systems

Educational Objectives

After reading Chapter 16 of the textbook and completing this exercise, the student will
1. Have a basic understanding and appreciation of the basic concepts of computer tomography (CT) scanning and magnetic resonance imaging (MRI).
2. Understand the role of CT and MRI in dentistry.

I. Definitions

Define/explain the following terms.

1. Axial plane _____

_____

2. Bone window _____

_____

3. Computed tomography (CT) _____

_____

4. CT number _____

_____

5. Digitize _____

_____

6. Electronic sensor _____

_____

7. Hounsfield unit (HU) _____

_____

8. Image acquisition _____

_____

9. Image reformatting _____

_____

10. Magnetic field _____

_____

11. Magnetic resonance imaging (MRI) _____

_____

12. Radiofrequency waves _____

_____

13. Signal intensity _____

_____

14. Soft tissue window _____

_____

15. Software _____

_____

II. Comprehension Exercise

1. What is the main difference between CT scanning and digital radiography?

2. Explain the advantage of using a CT scan instead of a panoramic film in the planning for implants.

3. What are the common themes employed between CT scanning and MRI?

4. What are CT numbers? Give an example.

5. Why is MRI a preferred method for imaging the articular disc of the temporomandibular joint (TMJ)?

6. Why has the "A" been dropped in "CAT" scan? What major change in the use of this technique is responsible for the alteration?

7. What is a weak signal?

8. What is the function of the powerful magnet in MRI?

9. Explain how a CT scan could be sent to the referring dentist.

10. What does image reformatting mean?

11. List five advantages of CT scanning.

12. How is tomography used in obtaining a CT scan?

13. Why is there no radiation risk to the patient with MRI?

14. List four disadvantages of CT scanning.

III. Matching

Match the items in *Column A* with the appropriate items in *Column B*.

Column A

_____ 1. CT number
_____ 2. sagittal cut
_____ 3. powerful magnet
_____ 4. proton density
_____ 5. strong signal
_____ 6. hard copy
_____ 7. radiofrequency waves
_____ 8. implant program
_____ 9. electronic detectors
_____ 10. information storage
_____ 11. software
_____ 12. weak signal
_____ 13. bone window
_____ 14. water content
_____ 15. zero Hounsfield units

Column B

a. directs the computer
b. hard tissue
c. Hounsfield units (HU)
d. signals to computer
e. 70% of the human body
f. high density
g. aligns protons
h. soft tissue
i. water
j. computer
k. MRI
l. resonance
m. given to the patient
n. long wavelengths
o. coronal plane
p. reformatted image
q. software

IV. Complete These Statements

1. For proper implant planning using CT scanning a special _____ is needed.

2. Seventy percent of the human body is _____.

3. CT was introduced into radiology in the early _____.

4. Radiofrequency waves and x-rays are part of the _____.

5. In CT scanning, the _____ is done in a tomographic mode with the detectors traveling 360 degrees around the patient.

6. In CT scanning, the computer collects the x-ray beam penetration data in a grid pattern called a _____.

7. A black area on an MR image indicates _____.

8. A new means to acquire the CT image is a technique called _____ _____ _____ using a two-dimensional x-ray sensor.

9. CT numbers range from _____ to _____.

10. Because radiofrequency energy waves are _____, they cannot cause ionization.

V. Multiple Choice

Select the best answer.

1. In MRI the powerful magnetic field in which the patient is placed
   a. causes ionization of tissue
   b. produces the signal
   c. generates the radiofrequency wave
   d. realigns the tissue protons
   e. all of the above

2. The CT image can be
   a. displayed on a monitor
   b. stored on a disk
   c. transmitted by phone to other locations
   d. reformatted in other planes
   e. all of the above

3. In CT the image is formed by the
   a. computer
   b. sensor
   c. tube movement
   d. magnetic field
   e. none of the above

4. Fat tissue has a Hounsfield unit value of
   a. +1000
   b. +100
   c. 0
   d. −1000
   e. none of the above

5. The views needed in a CT scan for implant evaluation are
   a. panoramic and coronal
   b. coronal
   c. sagittal
   d. axial and cross sectional
   e. all of the above

6. The main application of MRI in dentistry has been in imaging
   a. bone density
   b. the maxillary sinus
   c. the articular disc of the TMJ
   d. the mental foramen
   e. none of the above

7. The CT number for water is
   a. 0 Hu
   b. +1000 Hu
   c. −1000 Hu
   d. +117 Hu
   e. −50 Hu

8. In CT scanning, significant artifacts are produced by
   a. composite restorations
   b. metallic objects
   c. dense bone
   d. static electricity
   e. excessive bending

9. The radiation dose from a head scan is
   a. more than one conventional skull film
   b. the same as one skull film
   c. less than one skull film
   d. not comparable
   e. none of the above

10. The powerful magnetic field in MRI can lethally attract
    a. the operator
    b. the patient
    c. the water molecules
    d. the receptor
    e. any freestanding metal objects

VI. True/False

Select whether each statement is true (**T**) or false (**F**). Circle the correct answer.

1. CT scanning uses ionizing radiation as the energy source. **T/F**
2. Both CT scanning and MRI utilize the tomographic technique in image acquisition. **T/F**
3. Cone beam tomography produces equivalent radiation exposure to the patient when compared to medical CT scanning for dental use. **T/F**
4. Magnetic resonance imaging (MRI) utilizes microwave energy as its source. **T/F**
5. Soft tissues have a strong signal intensity on MRI images and appear as black areas. **T/F**

Chapter 17

Quality Assurance

I. Definitions

Define/explain the following terms.

1. AAOMR _____

_____

2. "Criteria for Intraoral Radiographs" _____

_____

3. Darkroom quality assurance program _____

_____

4. Lead contamination _____

_____

5. Lead-lined boxes _____

_____

6. "Longest in, first out" rule _____

_____

7. Protective devices _____

_____

8. Quality assurance program _____

_____

9. Reference film _____

_____

10. Step wedge _____

_____

II. Comprehension Exercise

1. What comprises the most critical part of the darkroom quality assurance program?

2. List the six categories for quality assurance named by the American Academy of Oral and Maxillofacial Radiology (AAOMR).

3. What items should be posted in the exposure and processing rooms?

4. List/explain two ways to check solution strength in a dental office.

5. Discuss the importance of a quality assurance program in the darkroom.

6. How can an office maintain high levels of chairside competence?

5. If clearing of a film requires more than 4 minutes, the fixer
   a. is too concentrated
   b. is too strong
   c. is acceptable for use
   d. will be fine after one week
   e. is too weak

6. Unexposed films should be stored at
   a. temperatures of 50 to 70° F and 40 to 60 percent relative humidity
   b. temperatures of 40 to 50° F and 30 to 40 percent relative humidity
   c. temperatures of 60 to 80° F and 0 to 70 percent relative humidity
   d. temperatures of 30 to 40° F and 50 to 60 percent relative humidity
   e. none of the above

7. The lead used to line the lead-lined boxes may oxidize and produce a white lead powder that is about
   a. 40% lead
   b. 70% lead
   c. 10% lead
   d. 50% lead
   e. 80% lead

8. For a darkroom quality assurance program to be effective
   a. the darkroom must be large enough to accommodate the staff
   b. the darkroom should be used for storage of film
   c. the viewbox in the darkroom should not be used
   d. the darkroom must be a darkroom and nothing else
   e. the thermometer does not have to be accurate

9. In order to use films before their expiration date, one should use
   a. the rule of "Selection Criteria"
   b. the "Criteria for Intraoral Radiographs"
   c. the "longest in, first out" rule
   d. the "maximum permissible dose"
   e. the "inverse square law"

10. It usually follows that developer and fixer solutions will need changing
   a. 1 week apart
   b. at the same time
   c. 2 to 3 weeks apart
   d. 2 days apart
   e. too often to perform the task at the same time

VI. True/False

Select whether each statement is true (**T**) or false (**F**). Circle the correct answer.

1. An effective quality assurance (QA) policy that monitors the use of x-radiation in a dental office is the sole responsibility of the dentist. **T/F**
2. Maintaining high levels of chairside competence is the basis of any successful QA program. **T/F**
3. The acronym "CRESO" stands for a Certified Radiation Equipment Safety Officer. **T/F**
4. The chemical strength and level of solutions in both manual tanks and automatic processors must be monitored on a weekly basis. **T/F**
5. Unexposed and unprocessed films, as well as solutions, should be stored in a cold, humid location. **T/F**

18

Patient Management and Special Problems

Educational Objectives

After reading Chapter 18 of the textbook and completing this exercise, the student will

1. Understand how to successfully relate to all patients in the dental environment.
2. Understand what special situations might arise in dental radiography and be able to deal with them clinically.
3. Be able to substitute alternative techniques in dental radiography when it is not possible to use the primary method.

I. Definitions

Define/explain the following terms.

1. Arthrography _____

_____

2. Buccal object rule _____

_____

3. Disability _____

_____

4. Gag reflex _____

_____

5. Localization by definition _____

_____

6. Marking grid _____

_____

7. Maxillary torus _____

_____

8. Measuring grid _____

_____

9. Radiopaque media _____

_____

10. Reverse bitewing _____

_____

11. Right-angle occlusal projection _____

_____

12. Sialography _____

_____

13. Three-plane localization _____

_____

14. Trismus _____

_____

15. Tube shift _____

_____

II. Comprehension Exercise

1. Explain the role of the dental professional in patient management.

2. Describe personal hygiene and infection control procedures in dental radiography of which the dental professional should be aware.

3. How has greeting a patient in the waiting room changed since the Health Information Privacy Accountability Act (HIPAA) legislation was initiated?

4. How can the dental professional convey a feeling of confidence to the patient?

5. What does one do when a patient refuses to have radiographs taken?

6. What will determine how the disabled patient is managed in the dental office?

7. Why is it important for the dental professional to be able to discuss radiation safety with the patient?

8. List and briefly describe some methods that may be used to prevent gagging.

9. What can the dental professional do if the pediatric patient does not cooperate while trying to take bitewing radiographs?

10. Describe three methods that can be used to localize an impaction.

11. What is the proper film order when taking a full-mouth radiographic survey? Why?

12. What techniques can the operator employ to facilitate placement of the mandibular anterior film when the lingual frenulum presents an anatomic constraint?

13. What are some clinical situations that may make it impossible to take intraoral radiographs?

14. List some methods that might be used to introduce a child to the use of dental x-rays.

15. Explain the use of the "same lingual, opposite buccal" (SLOB) rule in the tube shift localization technique.

III. Matching

Match the items in *Column A* with the appropriate items in *Column B*.

Column A

_____ 1. "show and tell"
_____ 2. radiopaque media
_____ 3. definition evaluation
_____ 4. arthrography
_____ 5. shallow palate
_____ 6. SLOB
_____ 7. reverse bitewing
_____ 8. right-angle occlusal
_____ 9. low palatal vault
_____ 10. gagging
_____ 11. grid
_____ 12. cuspid overlap
_____ 13. rubber dam
_____ 14. narrow arch
_____ 15. lingual frenulum

Column B

a. buccal object rule
b. lateral oblique
c. horizontal angulation
d. defensive reflex
e. change the film size
f. superimposed structures
g. temporomandibular joint (TMJ)
h. bisecting angle technique
i. gagging
j. sialogram
k. increased vertical angulation
l. tongue tied
m. pediatric curiosity
n. endodontic radiographs
o. topographic occlusal
p. localization
q. marking

IV. Illustrations

1. (Figure 18-1) Radiograph B was taken with an increased distal horizontal angulation from the initial radiograph A. Thus the foreign body must be:
   a. located buccally
   b. located lingually
   c. in a location that cannot be determined

_____

_____

_____

2. (Figure 18-2) What type of radiograph is this? What would be its use?

_____
_____
_____

V. Complete These Statements

1. In localization by definition, the object that is closest to the film has the better
   _____ .

2. In taking a full-mouth series, one should always start with the
   _____ .

3. _____ is a valuable tool in helping dental hygienists and assistants perform their chairside duties.

4. Suggestion, manner, and operator confidence are ways to prevent
   _____
   _____ .

5. To overcome maxillary cuspid overlap, the angulation is altered
   _____
   _____ .

6. One of the important roles of the dental professional is to try to
   _____
   _____ the patient, so that the work will be easier for everyone involved, including the patient.

7. Magnetic resonance imaging is particularly useful in dentistry in diagnosing pathologic processes of the
   _____ .

8. In endodontic radiography it is recommended that the rubber dam be
   _____
   _____ .

9. If a disabled patient is completely unmanageable, radiographs may have to be taken with the patient under
   _____ or
   _____ .

10. Soft tissue can be visualized or outlined on standard radiographs with the use of
    _____
    _____ .

11. Hand washing and gloving should always be done _____ of the patient.

12. The obvious challenge in treating the hearing impaired patient is
    _____
    _____ .

13. Two clinical situations where it may be impossible to take intraoral radiographs are _____ and _____.

14. Two methods that may be used to prevent patient gagging are _____ and _____.

15. Less than _____ % of dental patients have an impossibly sensitive gag reflex causing radiographic procedures to be completely intolerable.

VI. Multiple Choice

Select the best answer.

1. The gag reflex is
   a. an acquired habit
   b. not present in all patients
   c. a body defense mechanism
   d. a contraindication for intraoral radiography
   e. a reaction the operator can ignore

2. When a patient consistently moves the bitewing packet with the tongue and bites the packet, the operator should
   a. force the packet into position
   b. scold the patient
   c. hold the packet
   d. do a reverse bitewing
   e. take no bitewings

3. Dental professionals should never
   a. use localization techniques
   b. hold the film in a patient's mouth
   c. change the size of the film used
   d. use the bisecting technique
   e. explain the importance of dental radiographs to the patient

4. Proper patient management is the responsibility of the
   a. dentist
   b. hygienist
   c. dental assistant
   d. office manager
   e. all of the above

5. If an impacted third molar moves mesially on the second film when the horizontal angulation is increased distally, the impaction must be
   a. buccal
   b. on the crest of the ridge
   c. lingual
   d. horizontal
   e. vertical

6. The use of patient psychology to manage dental patients includes
   a. scheduling appointments
   b. screening telephone calls
   c. chairside responsibilities
   d. collecting fees
   e. all of the above

7. A shallow palate that will not allow proper placement of the film for the paralleling method
   a. is found very often
   b. never occurs
   c. is occasionally found
   d. requires that a panoramic film be taken
   e. requires that an occlusal film be taken

8. The lingual frenulum may
   a. present problems in radiographing the maxillary anteriors
   b. make it difficult to place the film parallel to the tooth
   c. prevent the bisecting method from being used
   d. not affect radiographic technique
   e. none of the above

9. Possible dental patient disabilities include all of the following *except*
   a. prominent mandibular tori
   b. hearing impairment
   c. physical disability
   d. vision impairment
   e. developmental disability

10. An impacted mandibular molar can be localized radiographically in the anterior posterior and superior inferior planes by taking
    a. a periapical film
    b. a panoramic film
    c. a lateral oblique film
    d. all of the above
    e. none of the above

11. Gagging in many cases can be controlled or prevented by
    a. general anesthesia
    b. use of undiluted mouthwash
    c. local anesthesia injection
    d. slower technique
    e. all of the above

12. In which dental specialty is the marking grid usually employed?
    a. prosthodontics
    b. periodontics
    c. pediatric dentistry
    d. orthodontics
    e. endodontics

13. In taking mandibular premolar periapical films, mandibular tori
    a. present severe problems using the paralleling method
    b. have no effect on the paralleling method
    c. restrict intraoral radiography to occlusal films
    d. necessitate the use of panoramic technique
    e. none of the above

14. Which of the following is probably the *least* reliable way to localize an impaction in the buccolingual plane?
    a. localization by definition
    b. maxillary right-angle occlusal
    c. right-angle mandibular occlusal
    d. buccal object rule
    e. none of the above

15. Sialography involves injecting radiopaque material into
    a. maxillary tori
    b. salivary glands and ducts
    c. the lingual frenulum
    d. the TMJ
    e. the ventral surface of the tongue

VII. True/False

Select whether each statement is true (**T**) or false (**F**). Circle the correct answer.

1. Patients must feel comfortable and confident about the dental professional's ability to perform the radiographic examination. **T/F**
2. Panoramic radiographs are useful with wheelchair-bound patients. **T/F**
3. Of all the problems one may encounter in intraoral radiography, gagging is probably the least troublesome. **T/F**
4. Structures that lie further from the x-ray film have better radiographic definition than those that lie closer to the film. **T/F**
5. The shallow palatal vault represents a problem in the paralleling technique. **T/F**

Chapter 19

Film Mounting and Radiographic Anatomy

Educational Objectives

After reading Chapter 19 of the textbook and completing this exercise, the student will

1. Understand what determines the radiographic appearance of teeth and the alveolar processes of the maxilla and mandible.
2. Recognize radiographic landmarks of the mandible and maxilla as seen on periapical and bitewing films.
3. Recognize normal radiographic anatomy seen on panoramic and occlusal films.

I. Definitions

Define/explain the following terms.

1. Curve of Spee _____

_____

2. Foramen _____

_____

3. Labial mounting _____

_____

4. Lingual mounting _____

_____

5. Orientation dot _____

_____

6. Radiographic anatomy _____

_____

7. Radiographic mount _____

_____

8. Radiolucent_____

_____

9. Radiopaque_____

_____

10. Sinus _____

_____

II. Comprehension Exercise

1. What determines whether an object or structure will be radiolucent or radiopaque?

2. Explain how to differentiate between a mandibular premolar and maxillary premolar film.

3. How does the orientation dot help to mount films in their correct anatomic position?

4. Which is the most radiopaque of all tooth structures?

5. Which is the most radiolucent of all tooth structures?

6. Why does the dental professional require a basic knowledge of radiographic anatomy in order to mount films correctly?

7. Radiographically, how can one differentiate mandibular molar edentulous films from maxillary molar edentulous films?

8. How and why do the lips, cheek, and tongue affect the radiograph?

9. What should be labeled on the mount to establish patient ownership of the radiographs?

10. On which extraoral projections can the maxillary sinus be seen? Which is the best view for visualizing the maxillary sinus?

11. On what intraoral projection is the coronoid process of the mandible seen?

12. How are bitewings mounted correctly?

13. Why is the mental foramen seen as a radiolucency?

14. Does the maxilla or the mandible have a denser trabecular pattern of bone? What is the clinical significance of this?

15. How can the dental professional distinguish between a foramen and a periapical pathologic process by means of radiographic interpretation alone?

III. Matching

Match the items in *Column A* with the appropriate items in *Column B*.

Column A

_____ 1. coronoid process
_____ 2. internal oblique ridge
_____ 3. lingual mounting
_____ 4. nasopalatine foramen
_____ 5. mandibular foramen
_____ 6. curve of Spee
_____ 7. labial mounting
_____ 8. cementum
_____ 9. zygomatic process of maxilla
_____ 10. nutrient canals
_____ 11. enamel
_____ 12. illuminator
_____ 13. greater radiation penetration
_____ 14. mental foramen
_____ 15. genial tubercle

Column B

a. vertical radiolucent lines
b. viewbox
c. lower incisor film
d. most radiopaque tooth structures
e. radiopaque covering on the root
f. not seen on a periapical survey
g. maxillary molar film
h. patient's right on viewer's left
i. mylohyoid ridge
j. mandibular condyle
k. U-shaped radiopacity
l. lower premolar film
m. maxillary incisor film
n. patient's left on viewer's left
o. radiolucent
p. bitewing radiographs
q. radiopaque band

IV. Illustrations

Identify the lettered structures on each of the following radiographs.

1. (Figure 19-1) Identify the labeled structures.

a. _____

b. _____

c. _____

d. _____

2. (Figure 19-2) Which intraoral radiographic projection is this? Assuming labial mounting, which side of the mouth is this? Identify the labeled structures.

a. _____

b. _____

c. _____

3. (Figure 19-3) Identify the following structures labeled A through F.

a. _____

b. _____

c. _____

d. _____

e. _____

f. _____

4. (Figure 19-4) Which intraoral radiographic projection is this? Identify the labeled structures.

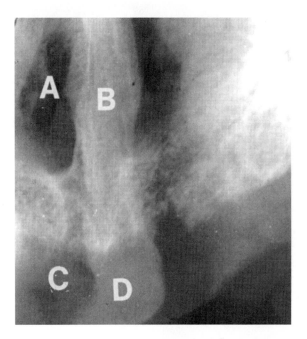

a. _____

b. _____

c. _____

d. _____

5. (Figure 19-5) Identify the labeled structures.

a. _____

b. _____

c. _____

6. (Figure 19-6) Identify structures A and B.

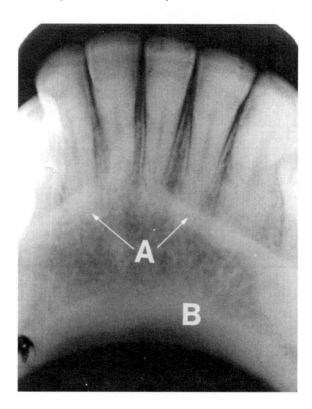

a. _____

b. _____

7. (Figure 19-7) Identify the labeled structures.

a. _____

b. _____

c. _____

d. _____

8. (Figure 19-8) Identify the labeled structures.

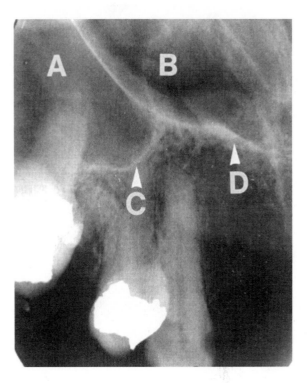

a. _____

b. _____

c. _____

d. _____

9. (Figure 19-9) Identify A and B.

a. _____

b. _____

10. (Figure 19-10) Identify A and B.

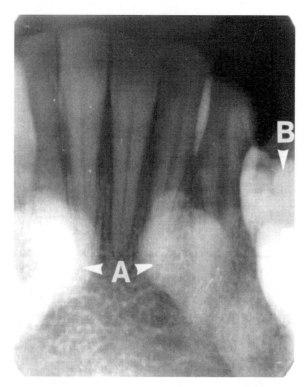

a. _____

b. _____

11. (Figure 19-11) What radiographic view is this? Assuming labial mounting, is it the patient's right or left? Identify the labeled structures.

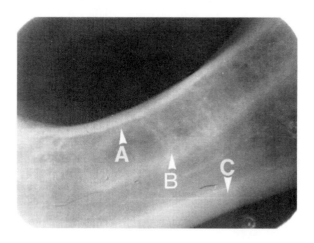

a. _____

b. _____

c. _____

12. (Figure 19-12) Identify the labeled structures.

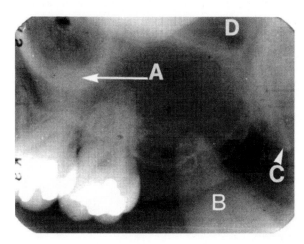

a. _____

b. _____

c. _____

d. _____

13. (Figure 19-13) Identify the labeled structures.

a. _____

b. _____

c. _____

d. _____

14. (Figure 19-14) Identify A and B.

a. _____

b. _____

15. (Figure 19-15) All teeth test vital. What is your interpretation of the radiolucency at the apex of the second premolar?

_____

_____

_____

16. (Figure 19-16) Assuming labial mounting, what side (left or right) and area does this radiograph show? Identify the labeled structures.

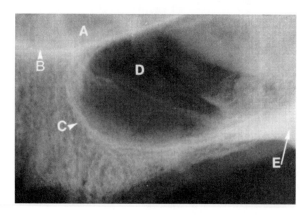

a. _____

b. _____

c. _____

d. _____

e. _____

17. (Figure 19-17) Identify the dense bony structure seen at the top of this radiograph.

_____

_____

18. (Figure 19-18) Identify the dense area of bone outlined by the arrows.

_____

_____

_____

V. Complete These Statements

1. The most universally accepted way to mount radiographs is the _____ method.

2. The mandibular canal can usually be seen on the _____ and periapical _____ radiographs.

3. When mounting it is important to remember that most roots curve _____.

4. The mental foramen, when it is superimposed on the apex of the premolar, can resemble _____.

5. The most radiopaque of all tooth structures is _____.

6. Cancellous bone radiographically is composed of small radiolucent compartments known as _____ separated by a radiopaque honeycomb pattern called _____.

7. A cement base under a deep restoration will appear _____ on a radiograph.

8. An acrylic crown will appear _____ on a radiograph.

9. The _____ is a depression in the labial plate in the maxillary lateral incisor area.

10. The nasal cavity may be seen on a _____ and a _____ periapical radiograph.

11. Roots of the maxillary molars can seem to be in the _____ when seen on radiographs.

12. The _____ is seen as a radiolucent area below the mylohyoid ridge.

13. Maxillary premolars usually have _____ root(s) whereas mandibular premolars have _____ root(s).

14. Metallic restorations will appear _____ on radiographs.

15. When interpreting occlusal films, the dental professional must remember that the projection is in the _____ plane.

VI. Multiple Choice

1. The periodontal ligament surrounding a normal tooth appears radiographically as
   a. an unbroken radiopaque line around the tooth root
   b. a radiopaque line on the lateral sides of the root
   c. an unbroken radiolucent line around the tooth root
   d. a radiolucent line around the apical portion only
   e. an unbroken radiolucent outline around the crown and root

2. Which of the following structures appear radiolucent on a radiograph?
   a. nares, median suture, medullary spaces
   b. incisive canal, genial tubercles, nasal fossa
   c. maxillary sinus, mylohyoid ridge, mental foramen
   d. hamular process, nutrient canals, nasal cartilage
   e. coronoid process, mandibular canal, maxillary septum

3. Which of the following is a major part of the tooth structure, appears radiopaque on radiographs, and is seen in both the crown and roots of the teeth?
   a. enamel
   b. cementum
   c. lamina dura
   d. dentin
   e. pulp

4. Which of the following anatomic structures is usually not demonstrated on intraoral periapical radiographs?
   a. mental foramen
   b. mylohyoid ridge
   c. coronoid process
   d. mandibular foramen
   e. median palatine suture

5. Arrange the following in order of increasing opacity
   a. dentin
   b. enamel
   c. amalgam
   d. zinc oxide–eugenol
   e. pulp
      (1) c, b, a, e, d
      (2) d, e, c, a, b
      (3) e, a, b, d, c
      (4) e, d, a, b, c

6. All of the following tooth structures appear radiopaque *except*
   a. enamel
   b. periodontal membrane
   c. lamina dura
   d. cementum
   e. dentin

7. Which of the following structures appear radiopaque on a radiograph?
   a. maxillary sinus, genial tubercle, nasal cavity
   b. nasal spine, external oblique ridge, mental foramen
   c. internal oblique ridge, median nasal septum, mental ridge
   d. inferior border of mandible, mental ridge, nares
   e. maxillary tuberosity, nasopalatine foramen, maxillary sinus

8. All of the following may be seen on a mandibular molar film *except*
   a. the mandibular canal
   b. the inferior border
   c. the condyle
   d. the internal oblique ridge
   e. the external oblique ridge

9. The occlusal part of the alveolar bone is referred to as the
   a. trabeculae
   b. lamina dura
   c. alveolar crest
   d. medullary spaces
   e. cancellous bone

10. Which of the following appears radiolucent on a radiograph?
    a. nasal turbinates
    b. nasal floor
    c. nasal septum
    d. nasal cavity
    e. nasal spine

11. All of the following may be seen on a maxillary premolar radiograph *except*
    a. the floor of the nose
    b. the buccinator shadow
    c. the maxillary sinus
    d. the maxillary tuberosity
    e. the zygomatic process of the maxilla

12. The radiolucent anatomic structure seen running vertically between the roots of the maxillary central incisors is the
    a. nasopalatine foramen
    b. incisive foramen
    c. nasal septum
    d. median palatine suture
    e. anterior nasal spine

13. Which of the following structures seen on a panoramic radiograph do not appear on an intraoral full-mouth survey?
    a. the inferior border of the mandible
    b. the maxillary tuberosity
    c. the coronoid process
    d. the hyoid bone
    e. the mandibular canal

14. The bilateral radiolucent band seen crossing the ascending ramus of the mandible on panoramic films represents
    a. the hard palate
    b. the soft palate
    c. the pharyngeal air space
    d. the nares
    e. the uvula

15. Which of the following can be seen on any mandibular radiograph?
    a. inferior border of the mandible
    b. external oblique ridge
    c. genial tubercles
    d. mental ridges
    e. mandibular canal

VII. True/False

Select whether each statement is true (**T**) or false (**F**). Circle the correct answer.

1. All radiographic structures appear either radiopaque (RO) or radiolucent (RL) without gradations in each category. **T/F**
2. Not all anatomic landmarks are always demonstrated on every full-mouth survey or individual films. **T/F**
3. It is not difficult to distinguish cementum from dentin on a radiograph. **T/F**
4. Most roots curve mesially. **T/F**
5. Nutrient canals are most easily seen in the mandibular anterior region. **T/F**

Chapter 20

Principles of Radiographic Interpretation

I. Definitions

Define/explain the following terms.

1. Anatomic landmark _____

_____

2. Benign lesion _____

_____

3. Bilateral lesion _____

_____

4. Differential diagnosis _____

_____

5. Interpretation _____

_____

6. Malignant lesion _____

_____

7. Radiolucent image _____

_____

8. Radiopaque image _____

_____

9. Unilateral lesion _____

_____

10. Vitality testing _____

_____

II. Comprehension Exercise

1. Why are the borders of a lesion important?

2. What are the three steps to be taken when interpreting dental radiographs?

3. What is considered advanced imaging?

4. Why is it important to the interpretation process for the dental professional to avoid committing technical exposure and processing errors?

5. When should a diagnostician order advanced studies?

6. Why should the dental professional ask a patient to reveal his or her chief complaint?

7. What is the importance of previous films?

8. What is the importance of seeing a suspicious oral lesion on three planes?

9. What is the significance of a lesion that appears bilaterally?

10. Why is it important to visualize dentulous as well as edentulous areas on radiographs?

III. Matching

Match the items in *Column A* with the appropriate items in *Column B*.

Column A	Column B
_____ 1. edentulous films	a. third-dimension visualization
_____ 2. anatomic landmarks	b. an explanation
_____ 3. buccal plate intact	c. located in the maxilla
_____ 4. horizontal overlap	d. identification of disease
_____ 5. root resorption	e. cyst
_____ 6. teeth movement	f. within normal limits
_____ 7. interpretation	g. benign lesion
_____ 8. distinct borders	h. faulty operator technique
_____ 9. median palatine cyst	i. should be taken
_____ 10. diagnosis	j. malignancy
	k. advanced imaging
	l. periapical radiograph

IV. Complete These Statements

1. Previous films are important because they
   _____
   _____.

2. To produce adequate diagnostic films, the operator should know
   _____
   _____.

3. Most bone lesions are
   _____.

4. Approximately
   _____ % of all pathologic oral conditions are the result of nonvital teeth.

5. One must see all of the
   _____ of a lesion.

6. _____ are located in very specific areas in the oral cavity and are diagnostically within normal limits.

7. Poorly defined borders of a lesion are usually seen in
   _____ lesions.

8. A lesion is considered
   _____ if it has one compartment and _____ if there is more than one compartment.

9. An area that is _____ should be radiographed in order to examine the area for impaction, unerupted teeth, and bone pathologic processes.

10. Rapidly growing lesions that do not have distinct borders are usually
    _____ lesions.

V. Multiple Choice

Select the best answer.

1. An example of an anatomic landmark resembling a periapical pathology (PAP) is the
   a. zygomatic arch
   b. nasopalatine foramen
   c. internal oblique ridge
   d. external oblique ridge
   e. anterior nasal spine

2. The interpretation of radiographs primarily provides the basis for building a
   a. chief complaint
   b. diagnosis
   c. prevention plan
   d. treatment plan
   e. dental history

3. The patient's chief complaint may be
   a. swelling
   b. pain
   c. loose teeth
   d. bleeding
   e. all of the above

4. Which of the following is *not* a step that is to be taken in building a diagnosis?
   a. interpretation of what has been identified
   b. identification of an area or structure that is questionable
   c. diagnosis based on the interpretation
   d. extraction of a tooth that is symptomatic
   e. distinguishing an anatomic landmark from a pathologic lesion

5. A dental professional may want to use CT scanning
   a. for visualizing the articulator disc
   b. for cross-sectional views
   c. for evaluating previous fillings
   d. instead of a panoramic radiograph
   e. to evaluate the overlapping of teeth

6. Dental professionals should develop the skills to
   a. identify all normal anatomy
   b. identify tooth structure
   c. identify bone structure
   d. identify artifacts
   e. all of the above

7. A rapidly growing, radiolucent lesion with irregular borders in the oral cavity could be a sign of
   a. a cyst
   b. an infectious lesion
   c. a devitalized defect
   d. a malignancy
   e. an anatomic landmark

8. Possible pathologic lesions should be described by
   a. size
   b. tooth movement
   c. bone resorption
   d. root resorption
   e. all of the above

9. Most lesions in the oral cavity are
   a. radiopaque
   b. radiolucent
   c. both radiolucent and radiopaque
   d. it depends on whether it is within normal limits or not
   e. only visible on panoramic radiographs

10. Other signs and symptoms that can be used in establishing a diagnosis along with radiographic interpretation are
    a. the patient's chief complaint
    b. biopsy
    c. medical history
    d. clinical examination
    e. all of the above

VI. True/False

Select whether each statement is true (**T**) or false (**F**). Circle the correct answer.

1. Interpretation of the radiographs is the only step necessary in formulating a diagnosis. **T/F**
2. To produce adequate diagnostic films, the dental professional must know what relevant information is being sought from the radiograph. **T/F**
3. About 70% of all pathologic conditions seen in the jaws are the result of nonvital teeth and their sequelae. **T/F**
4. Most bilateral findings are normal anatomic landmarks. **T/F**
5. Malignant lesions tend to grow slowly. **T/F**

Chapter

21

Caries and Periodontal Disease

Educational Objectives

After reading Chapter 21 of the textbook and completing this exercise, the student will

1. Understand the effect of caries and periodontal disease on the radiographic appearance of teeth and alveolar bone.
2. Be able to recognize caries on radiographs, correlate clinical findings with radiographic findings, differentiate caries from anatomic features and restorative materials, and be able to judge the extent of caries.
3. Be able to recognize the limitations of radiographs in caries detection.
4. Be able to recognize the signs of periodontal disease on radiographs.
5. Be able to diagnose the extent of bone loss and identify predisposing factors.

I. Definitions

Define/explain the following terms.

1. Abrasion_____

_____

2. Advanced caries _____

_____

3. Attrition_____

_____

4. Carious exposure _____

_____

5. Cemento-enamel junction _____

_____

6. Cervical burnout _____

_____

7. Composite filling material _____

_____

8. Gingivitis _____

_____

9. Incipient caries _____

_____

10. Indirect pulp capping _____

_____

11. Interproximal bone loss _____

_____

12. Interproximal overlapped film _____

_____

13. Occlusal caries _____

_____

14. Periodontal disease _____

_____

15. Pulpotomy _____

_____

II. Comprehension Exercise

1. Explain the role of the dental professional in dental diagnosis.

2. Give an example of how an error in radiographic technique can lead to a deficient diagnosis.

3. Explain how caries appears on radiographs initially and as it progresses.

4. Why does caries appear radiolucent on radiographs?

5. Name some conditions found on radiographs that might be misinterpreted as caries.

6. What is the best way to detect occlusal caries?

7. Why is it difficult to see buccal or lingual caries on radiographs?

8. Name some predisposing factors to periodontal disease that can be seen on radiographs.

9. What oral conditions are bitewing radiographs especially useful in detecting?

10. Describe the appearance of calculus on radiographs. Is it always seen radiographically?

11. Why are buccal and lingual caries difficult to detect on radiographs?

12. What are the radiographic signs of early periodontal disease?

13. What are the radiographic signs of advanced periodontal disease?

14. What radiographic exposure technique is preferred for identifying periodontal disease radiographically? Explain.

15. Explain the radiographic finding of "cervical burnout."

III. Matching

Match the items in *Column A* with the appropriate items in *Column B*.

Column A

_____ 1. periodontal ligament space
_____ 2. resembles periapical pathology
_____ 3. lamina dura
_____ 4. bisecting technique
_____ 5. nonpenetration of photons
_____ 6. calculus
_____ 7. not seen on radiographs
_____ 8. early periodontal disease
_____ 9. radiolucent
_____ 10. advanced periodontal disease
_____ 11. short roots
_____ 12. photons penetrate object
_____ 13. interproximal caries
_____ 14. mistaken for caries
_____ 15. poor way to see caries

Column B

a. radiopaque
b. triangulation
c. bifurcation involvement
d. thin radiolucent line
e. buccal caries
f. cervical burnout
g. gingivitis
h. radiolucent
i. bitewing film
j. thin radiopaque line
k. panoramic films
l. etiologic factor for periodontitis
m. dimensional distortion
n. mental foramen
o. poor prognosis
p. acrylic
q. occlusal film

IV. Illustrations

1. (Figure 21-1) Identify the caries on this radiograph.

_____

_____

_____

2. (Figure 21-2) Identify the caries on this radiograph.

_____

_____

3. (Figure 21-3) How would you classify the periodontal bone condition on this radiograph?

_____

_____

_____

4. (Figure 21-4) What periodontal conditions appear on this radiograph?

_____

_____

_____

5. (Figure 21-5) Differentiate between the cervical radiolucencies seen on the mesial and distal surfaces of the first molar. How would you confirm your radiographic diagnosis?

_____

_____

_____

6. (Figure 21-6) What is your interpretation of the radiolucent area seen on the mesial of the canine (cuspid)?

_____

_____

_____

7. (Figure 21-7) Identify the caries, if any, on this radiograph.

_____

_____

_____

8. (Figure 21-8) What type of periodontal bone change appears on this radiograph?

_____

_____

_____

9. (Figure 21-9) Locate the calculus on this radiograph.

_____

_____

_____

10. (Figure 21-10) Locate the caries on this radiograph.

_____

_____

_____

11. (Figure 21-11) How would you classify the periodontal condition shown here? What is the prognosis?

_____

_____

_____

12. (Figure 21-12) Identify the caries in this radiograph.

_____

_____

_____

13. (Figure 21-13) Identify the radiopaque area pointed out by the arrow.

_____

_____

_____

V. Complete These Statements

After the following terms, record whether they appear radiopaque (RO) or radiolucent (RL) on radiographs.

1. amalgam filling _____

2. lamina dura _____

3. periodontal ligament space _____

4. old composite restoration _____

5. indirect pulp capping _____

6. caries _____

7. pulp chamber _____

8. mental foramen _____

9. infrabony pocket _____

10. alveolar bone _____

11. porcelain crown _____

12. pulp canal _____

13. cement base under filling _____

14. cervical abrasion _____

15. calculus _____

VI. Multiple Choice

Select the best answer.

1. The best intraoral radiographic projection for detecting caries is
   a. the bitewing
   b. periapical using the paralleling technique
   c. panoramic
   d. a and b
   e. all of the above

2. Radiographic changes evident in gingivitis include
   a. a widened lamina dura
   b. loss of interdental supporting bone
   c. furcation involvement
   d. both a and b
   e. none of the above

3. The most common reason for taking dental radiographs is the detection of
   a. horizontal bone loss
   b. vertical bone loss
   c. caries
   d. faulty restorations
   e. none of the above

4. The most likely diagnosis of an interproximal radiolucency just above the cervical line on a clinically caries-negative tooth is
   a. incipient caries
   b. attrition
   c. erosion
   d. cervical burnout
   e. none of the above

5. It is difficult to visualize buccal caries radiographically because
   a. the x-ray photons do not penetrate
   b. of overlying normal structures
   c. of increased density
   d. of decreased density
   e. none of the above

6. Calcified supragingival calculus on the lingual surfaces of teeth is not seen clearly on a radiograph because
   a. it is more detectable on the buccal surface
   b. of superimposition of tooth structure
   c. it is radiolucent
   d. it is not necessary for periodontal diagnosis
   e. all of the above

7. Gingival recession is not detectable radiographically because
   a. the angulation is wrong
   b. soft tissue is not seen
   c. the recession is out of the field
   d. an increased kVp would be needed
   e. none of the above

8. Cup-shaped bony defects are seen radiographically in
   a. the early stages of periodontal disease
   b. the advanced stages of periodontal disease
   c. the stage of periodontal disease associated with abscesses only
   d. early gingivitis
   e. none of the above

9. When caries invades the dentin from the enamel, it is seen as
   a. a radiopacity
   b. advancing straight toward the pulp
   c. spreading laterally and then advancing toward the pulp
   d. calcifying
   e. none of the above

10. As for periodontal prognosis, teeth that have anatomically short roots will
    a. have a poorer prognosis
    b. have a better prognosis
    c. be more resistant
    d. be less resistant
    e. none of the above

11. The infrabony pocket is seen with
    a. horizontal bone loss
    b. gingivitis
    c. poor crown-root ratio
    d. vertical bone loss
    e. none of the above

12. The crown-root ratio as seen on radiographs becomes critical in
    a. caries detection
    b. the choice of amalgam or composite for restorations
    c. designating abutments for a fixed bridge
    d. periodontal probing
    e. none of the above

13. In the clinical setting, caries seen radiographically is almost always
    a. less advanced
    b. missing
    c. further advanced
    d. calcified
    e. none of the above

14. The type of caries best detected on radiographs is
    a. occlusal caries
    b. buccal caries
    c. cervical caries
    d. interproximal caries
    e. none of the above

15. All of the following can resemble caries radiographically *except*
    a. attrition
    b. abrasion
    c. amalgam restorations
    d. composite restorations
    e. none of the above

VII. True/False

Select whether each statement is true (**T**) or false (**F**). Circle the correct answer.

1. Detection of caries is probably the most common reason for taking dental radiographs. **T/F**
2. Incipient caries is not difficult to detect radiographically. **T/F**
3. The first radiographic sign of interproximal caries is a notching of the enamel, usually just below the contact point. **T/F**
4. Evaluating the width of the periodontal ligament space is an important component of a radiographic periodontal examination. **T/F**
5. Triangulation of the periodontal membrane is seen radiographically in the advanced stages of periodontal disease. **T/F**

Chapter

22

Pulpal and Periapical Lesions

Educational Objectives

After reading Chapter 22 of the textbook and completing this exercise, the student will
1. Understand the process and sequelae of pulp necrosis and its radiographic findings.
2. Be able to diagnose radiographically periapical pathology and differentiate between it and normal anatomy as well as other apical findings.

I. Definitions

Define/explain the following terms.

1. Condensing osteitis _____

_____

2. Dentoalveolar abscess _____

_____

3. External resorption _____

_____

4. Internal resorption _____

_____

5. Periapical cemental dysplasia (PCD) (Periapical cemental osseous dysplasia [PCOD])

_____

_____

6. Periapical cyst _____

_____

7. Periapical granuloma _____

_____

8. Periapical pathology _____

_____

9. Pulp calcification _____

_____

10. Pulp denticle _____

_____

11. Pulpitis _____

_____

12. Residual cyst _____

_____

13. Residual granuloma _____

_____

14. Root resorption _____

_____

15. Secondary dentin _____

_____

II. Comprehension Exercise

1. Explain why vital and nonvital pulp can appear the same on a radiograph.

2. List the causative factors of pulpal necrosis that can be seen on radiographs.

3. List three causes for a change in the normal size and shape of the pulp chamber and canals.

4. What is the first radiographic finding other than etiologic factors of periapical pathology?

5. How can you differentiate between periapical pathology and PCD (PCOD)?

6. What is secondary dentin, and what is its appearance and clinical significance?

7. What are the most common causes for the formation of secondary dentin?

8. How can you differentiate radiographically between internal and external idiopathic root resorption?

9. What tissues are affected by periapical pathology?

10. Describe the radiographic appearance of condensing osteitis. How does it differ from cementoma (PCD)?

11. Why are periapical cysts seen as radiolucencies?

12. In making a diagnosis of a necrotic pulp, why is it essential to see the apex of the tooth on the radiograph?

13. Name some possible causes of root resorption.

14. What are the radiographic signs of pulpitis?

15. Explain the progression of PCD (PCOD) and how it appears radiographically in all three stages.

III. Matching

Match the items in *Column A* with the appropriate items in *Column B*.

Column A

_____ 1. secondary dentin
_____ 2. condensing osteitis
_____ 3. calcified pulp
_____ 4. root resorption
_____ 5. three-stage lesion
_____ 6. internal resorption
_____ 7. pulp denticle
_____ 8. periapical pathology
_____ 9. fistulous tract
_____ 10. external root resorption
_____ 11. high pulp horns
_____ 12. residual cyst
_____ 13. periapical cyst
_____ 14. pulpitis
_____ 15. decrease in pulp size

Column B

a. seen in young patients
b. pulpal tissue resorbs the dentin
c. vertical bone loss
d. exudate spills from the pulp
e. difficult to see on radiographs
f. pulp stone
g. present in edentulous areas
h. no radiographic sign
i. PCD (PCOD)
j. dentinogenesis imperfecta
k. no treatment indicated
l. radiolucent
m. idiopathic
n. hard to distinguish
o. agenesis
p. may be asymptomatic
q. chronic infection

IV. Illustrations

1. (Figure 22-1) There is pain and tenderness in the mucobuccal fold in the area of the extracted central incisor. All teeth test vital. What is your diagnosis?

_____

_____

_____

2. (Figure 22-2) This radiograph was taken of an asymptomatic new patient. What is your diagnosis for the condition seen here?

_____

_____

_____

3. (Figure 22-3) What is your diagnosis for this condition seen in this 49-year-old woman where all teeth test vital?

_____

_____

_____

4. (Figure 22-4) The lower first molar is nonvital. What is your diagnosis of the radiopacity on the distal root?

_____

_____

_____

5. (Figure 22-5) Pain and swelling are associated with the lateral incisor. What is your diagnosis?

_____

_____

_____

3. (Figure 24-3) What is your interpretation of the radiopaque structure seen here?

_____

_____

_____

4. (Figure 24-4) This patient fell off a bicycle, sustaining lacerations to the lip and cheek. The cuspid is extremely painful to touch. What is your diagnosis?

_____

_____

5. (Figure 24-5) Give two possible diagnoses for the radiopaque area the arrow is pointing to in this illustration.

_____

_____

_____

V. Complete These Statements

1. A sialolith of the submandibular duct can best be seen on a _____ radiographic projection.

2. Salivary stones are a common cause of _____, _____, and _____.

3. An intraosseous tumor that has the density of tooth components is an _____.

4. Three projections for viewing a sialolith in the parotid gland are a _____, _____, and a _____ placed in the mucobuccal fold.

5. Intraosseous malignant tumors will usually _____ the buccal cortex of the jawbones.

6. Retained root tips have the density of _____, making them difficult to differentiate from dense areas of bone.

7. An example of a radiopaque benign tumor is a _____.

8. Only those foreign bodies that are _____ can be seen radiographically.

9. The extraoral projection that is used to visualize the cottonwool appearance in Paget's disease is the _____.

10. Tooth and root fractures can lead to pulp damage and ensuing _____ conditions.

11. The radiopaque line seen on radiographs surrounding a slow-growing tumor is called the _____.

12. In a suspected fracture of the mandible the two radiographic projections that should be taken are the _____ and the _____.

13. An extraction socket is usually filled in with bone in about _____.

14. A tumor that tends to move teeth is usually _____.

15. An unerupted tooth surrounded by a large radiolucent area is usually the description of a _____.

VI. Multiple Choice

Select the best answer.

1. Which of the following pathologic conditions appears radiopaque on intraoral radiographs?
   a. a granuloma
   b. a periapical cyst
   c. an osteoma
   d. a connective tissue tumor
   e. none of the above

2. Tumors can appear
   a. radiolucent
   b. radiopaque
   c. mixed
   d. any of the above are possible
   e. a and b only

3. The buccal and lingual cortex surrounding a tumor of the mandible can best be seen on a
   a. panoramic radiograph
   b. topographic occlusal film
   c. lateral oblique projection
   d. right-angle occlusal projection
   e. none of the above

4. The radiographic differentiation between a retained root tip and a dense area of bone often can be done by identifying
   a. enamel
   b. cementum
   c. dentin
   d. a pulp canal
   e. none of the above

5. Metabolic radiographic bone lesions can be seen with
   a. Paget's disease
   b. types of anemia
   c. hyperparathyroidism
   d. any of the above is possible
   e. none of the above

6. The trabecular pattern of bone in a suspected metabolic lesion can best be interpreted with
   a. bitewing film
   b. periapical film
   c. panoramic film
   d. extraoral film
   e. none of the above

7. In making a radiographic diagnosis of a suspected tumor
   a. all the borders of the lesion must be seen
   b. the distal border must be seen
   c. the buccal cortex must be seen
   d. the center of the lesion must be seen
   e. none of the above

8. Extraction sockets are initially seen as
   a. radiolucent areas
   b. radiopaque areas
   c. mixed areas
   d. any of the above are possible
   e. a and b only

9. Fractures of the mandible or maxilla may appear radiographically as
   a. a radiopaque line
   b. a radiolucent line
   c. a radiolucent area
   d. a mixed area
   e. none of the above

10. A sialolith in the parotid gland can be seen in a
    a. lateral oblique projection
    b. posteroanterior projection
    c. soft tissue film placed in the mucobuccal fold
    d. CT scan
    e. all of the above

11. When radiographed, all suspected tumors must be viewed
    a. buccally
    b. lingually
    c. occlusally
    d. in all three planes
    e. none of the above

12. On a radiograph an amalgam fragment in an extraction socket will appear
    a. radiopaque
    b. not at all
    c. radiolucent
    d. part radiolucent, part radiopaque
    e. none of the above

13. A common cause of dry mouth, swelling, and pain under the tongue, especially after eating, is a(n)
    a. odontoma
    b. periapical cyst
    c. sialolith
    d. periapical abscess
    e. none of the above

14. Which of the following projections will be diagnostic for the buccal and lingual cortex of the mandible?
    a. panoramic
    b. periapical
    c. lateral oblique
    d. posterior anterior
    e. none of the above

15. The best radiograph for viewing a sialolith in the submandibular gland is
    a. a right-angle mandibular occlusal projection
    b. a topographic mandibular occlusal projection
    c. a topographic maxillary occlusal projection
    d. a right-angle maxillary occlusal projection
    e. none of the above

VII. True/False

Select whether each statement is true (**T**) or false (**F**). Circle the correct answer.

1. Malignancies tend to have poorly defined radiographic borders and destroy normal anatomic structures. **T/F**

2. Many metabolic conditions manifest themselves with changes of the trabecular pattern and lamina dura of bone in the mandible and maxilla. **T/F**

3. Fractures of teeth, especially anterior teeth, are very uncommon. **T/F**

4. Retained root tips do not have the density of tooth structure and are easily distinguished from dense areas of bone. **T/F**

5. Stones in the parotid gland can best be seen on mandibular occlusal film. **T/F**

Chapter

25

Legal Considerations

Educational Objectives

After reading Chapter 25 of the textbook and completing this exercise, the student will
1. Understand the laws and regulations that govern the use of radiation in dentistry.

I. Definitions

Define/explain the following terms.

1. Confidentiality _____

_____

2. Direct supervision _____

_____

3. General supervision _____

_____

4. Informed consent _____

_____

5. Liability _____

_____

6. Licensure _____

_____

7. Radiation inspections _____

_____

8. Respondeat superior _____

_____

9. Risk management _____

_____

10. Statute of limitations _____

_____

II. Comprehension Exercise

1. Is it acceptable for the insurance company to request preoperative and postoperative radiographs on a patient? Explain.

2. How long should dental radiographs be kept for a patient after he or she has ceased being a patient in the office?

3. How long does an adult patient have to file a lawsuit after the injury is committed? How long if the patient is a child?

4. Who owns the radiographic series—the patient or the dentist? What rights to the radiographs does the patient have? Explain.

5. What confidentiality issues apply to dental radiographs as a permanent part of a patient's records?

6. Why is it vitally important to keep accurate patient records?

7. What is risk management and who should participate in the program in a dental office?

8. Why is it important for the dental support staff to review the patient's health history before taking radiographs?

9. What is the difference between direct and general supervision in a dental office and how are these principles applied to dental radiography?

10. In what three major categories are the legal considerations regarding the use of ionizing radiation in dentistry included?

III. Matching

Match the items in *Column A* with the appropriate items in *Column B*.

Column A

_____ 1. risk management
_____ 2. direct supervision
_____ 3. respondeat superior
_____ 4. negligent
_____ 5. general supervision
_____ 6. full disclosure
_____ 7. informed consent
_____ 8. res gestae
_____ 9. standard of care
_____ 10. HIPAA

Column B

a. captain of the ship principle
b. admissions against interest
c. permission granted
d. dentist is physically present
e. at fault
f. confidentiality
g. personal radiation exposure
h. ownership of radiographs
i. dentist can be reached
j. reduce likelihood of suits
k. informing the patient
l. statute of limitations
m. usually performed procedures

IV. Complete These Statements

1. The _____ is the guardian of the dental radiographs.

2. The three most important parts of a defense in a malpractice suit are the "_____, _____, and _____."

3. The statute of limitation for an adult patient to file suit is _____ years and for a child it is approximately _____ years after he or she has reached the age of 21.

4. The insurance company cannot request _____ radiographs because their use is considered administrative.

5. All radiographic equipment manufactured or sold after _____ must meet federal regulations.

6. Many states require biannual or triennial _____ of the x-ray machines in the dental office.

7. _____ is the policies and procedures designed to reduce the likelihood of suits for malpractice against dentists.

8. _____, professionally and legally, rests with the dentist and not the dental hygienist or the dental assistant.

9. _____ means that the dentist is physically present in the office when the radiographs are being taken by the dental hygienist or assistant.

10. Radiographs of poor _____ can weaken the defense in a lawsuit for which they are being used as evidence.

V. Multiple Choice

Select the best answer.

1. Ownership of the radiographs rests with the
   a. dentist
   b. hygienist
   c. patient
   d. assistant
   e. none of the above

2. Insurance carriers can request
   a. postoperative radiographs
   b. preoperative radiographs
   c. any radiograph taken on the patient
   d. only the patient's radiographs that were taken during the last year
   e. none of the above

3. The dental office supportive staff can participate in obtaining informed consent from the patient, which entails
   a. formulating a diagnosis
   b. formulating a prognosis
   c. explaining the nature and purpose of the procedure to the patient
   d. holding back any information about the procedures to the patient
   e. none of the above

4. The doctrine of respondeat superior is also known as the
   a. res gestae
   b. "captain of the ship" principle
   c. risk management theory
   d. statute of limitations
   e. none of the above

5. The legal considerations with which dental assistants and hygienists should be concerned regarding the dental use of ionizing radiation are
   a. regulations regarding x-ray equipment
   b. risk management
   c. licensure and periodic inspection for users of x-ray equipment
   d. a and b only
   e. all of the above

6. Statements made by anyone at the time of an alleged negligent act are
   a. not admissible as evidence
   b. only admissible as evidence if recorded
   c. only admissible as evidence if repeated
   d. admissible as evidence
   e. none of the above

7. Dental radiographs are considered a part of the patient's dental record and are therefore considered
   a. to be illegal documents
   b. to be negligible documents
   c. to be liable documents
   d. to be legal documents
   e. none of the above

8. If the radiographic evidence presented to the court is illegible, the court may
   a. request the original radiographs
   b. not accept the radiographs as evidence
   c. allow the case to be affected by the lack of evidence
   d. a and b only
   e. all of the above

9. Dental procedures should not be performed without current and diagnostic radiographs because their use is now
   a. the only dental records needed for diagnosis
   b. the standard of care
   c. the only dental record needed for insurance purposes
   d. the only dental record needed to formulate a prognosis
   e. none of the above

10. The patient's records are
    a. discussed freely among dental professionals
    b. discussed only with the dental hygienist
    c. discussed only with the dentist
    d. confidential
    e. none of the above

VI. True/False

Select whether each statement is true (**T**) or false (**F**). Circle the correct answer.

1. All dental x-ray machines either manufactured or sold in the United States after 1974 must meet the federal government's performance standards. **T/F**
2. The dental professional should be knowledgeable about the rules and regulations of the state in which he or she is exposing radiographs. **T/F**
3. Liability, both professionally and legally, rests with all members of the dental staff. **T/F**
4. Dental radiographs are considered part of the patient's dental record but are not considered legal documents. **T/F**
5. The contents or findings in the patient's records are strictly confidential and should never be discussed or shown to anyone outside the dental facility. **T/F**